Developing Holistic Education
A Case Study of Raddery School for Emotionally Damaged Children

Philip Seed

Illustrations by Christopher Fry

Foreword

by

Sir Kenneth Alexander

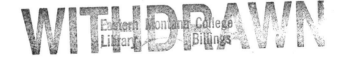
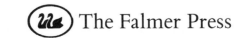 The Falmer Press

(A member of the Taylor & Francis Group)
London • Washington, D.C.

UK   The Falmer Press, 4 John St., London WC1N 2ET
USA   The Falmer Press, Taylor & Francis Inc., 1900 Frost Road, Suite 101,
        Bristol, PA 19007

First published 1992

A Catalogue record for this book is available from the British Library

Library of Congress Cataloging-in-Publication Data are available on request

ISBN 0 75070 060 2 cased
Cover Design by Caroline Archer

Set in 12/14pt Bembo
by Graphicraft Typesetters Ltd., Hong Kong

Printed in Great Britain by Burgess Science Press, Basingstoke on paper which has a specified pH value on final paper manufacture of not less than 7·5 and is therefore 'acid free'.

Contents

Foreword   vii
Sir Kenneth Alexander

Chapter 1   Introduction — A Very Special School for   1
             Children with Very Special Needs

Part I: The Raddery Experience   9

Chapter 2   Raddery as a Community   11

Chapter 3   Raddery as a School   41

Chapter 4   The Raddery Experience Viewed by Children,   65
             Parents and Staff

Chapter 5   Raddery in Context   107

Part II: Policy and Practice Implications   139

Chapter 6   Residential Child Care   141

Chapter 7   Special Education   153

Chapter 8   Preparation for Inter dependent Living   165

Chapter 9   Return to Raddery and Summary of   175
             Conclusions

Index   185

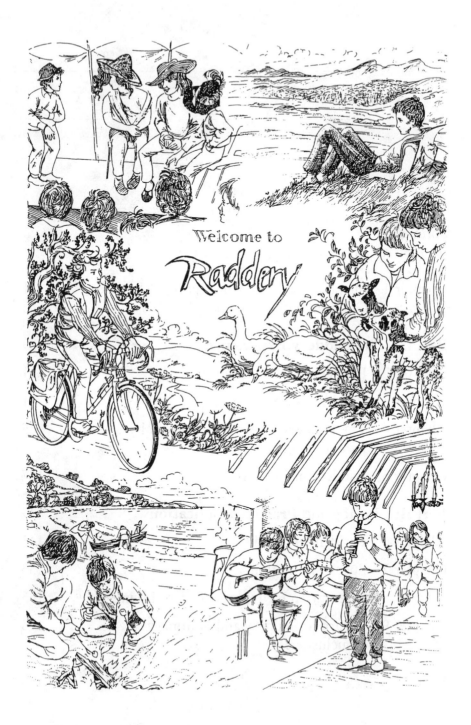

Welcome to Raddery

Foreword

The educational needs of emotionally damaged children and the existing provisions for these children are unchartered territory for a substantial majority of the general public and not widely understood, either, amongst most educationists. This book provides us with information and understanding on this very important aspect of education.

The book is a case study of Raddery School written by an academic who has had a close relationship with the school since its foundation ten years ago. The author brings to the study a great deal of relevant experience which enables him to make useful links and comparisons with alternative approaches to the educational challenge faced by all schools in this specialist area. The book avoids tedious description and makes the work at Raddery come alive on the page.

The concept of holistic education is explained and illustrated in many examples. It goes beyond John Stuart Mill's prescription for sound education that 'mind must be taught by mind' to recognize the need to build on spiritual foundations, build a sense of community with the whole infused by love.

Raddery is residential with very favourable staff to pupil ratios. A great deal of effort and attention is given to involving parents, and to a certain extent the school provides an extension or supplement to the family. Clearly, resources in ordinary non-residential schools cannot match those available at Raddery, but it is worth considering whether the philosophy of holistic education could be developed more widely. Just as at Raddery where the level of disturbance and damage which is brought to the school appears to have increased, so in the wider world heightening tensions and stresses suggest that more dimensions rather than narrower specialization could bring social as well as educational benefits.

Issues raised in this book will be of great interest to teachers. The problem of establishing and exercising authority within a very democratic structure, when difficult decisions have to be taken — on how to respond to crisis situations with pupils, on how to bring about necessary changes in established structures, or, more generally, how to move the school up its own learning curve in what was essentially an experimental situation. A network of similar schools has been established, creating opportunities to learn from each other, again involving discussion, the search for the correct answer and the best means of adjusting to the perceived need for change.

Despite Philip Seed's involvement with Raddery, he demonstrates a capacity for critical assessment of the school, illustrated by his 'thinking aloud' about various aspects of its life. I found no difficulty in trusting his judgement when he reaches very favourable conclusions on a range of the school's achievements. He writes '... at the deepest spiritual level, the act of love is complete in itself. This does not abrogate the responsibility to examine methods and goals. But the testimony of effective understanding and care, as a method and as a goal — as the means and the end — rather than a search for "smooth" progress, is ultimately the yardstick of any "success".' If the spirit and the practice behind such an approach can be created and sustained the lives of individual pupils and the communities in which they settle will be greatly enhanced.

The book has an additional attraction in the heart-warming illustrations by Christopher Fry.

Kenneth Alexander
February 1992

Chapter 1

Introduction — A Very Special School for Children with Very Special Needs

At one level, this book is about the care and education of children with very special needs. The needs result from emotional damage which impinges on their lives both at school and at home. At another level it is about the development of a holistic approach to education — applicable to children generally.

The first part of the book describes the Raddery experience. Raddery was established in the North of Scotland in 1979 as a voluntary-run school with charitable status. It is one of a number of special schools based on a holistic and therapeutic community approach. It comprises forty children and about the same number of staff adults. There are five to six children in each class and for children needing very individualized and personal attention in an informal setting there is a 'foundation unit'. Education throughout the day and evening, seven days a week, encompasses an enormous range of activities, appealing to every aspect of each child's potential. A therapeutic approach underpins education and is, in turn, promoted through education. Five living units called 'venues', where children spend much of their domestic time together, are separately located in three different parts of the main building, in a nearby cottage and (for some older children who have made substantial progress) in a separate house in a village a few miles away. Yet the emphasis is on 'one community' which finds specific expression in intensive staff support, a complex network of community meetings, and a daily morning meeting. There is a major emphasis on children learning together and supporting one another with the care, help and understanding of staff. In summary, education, care and therapy take place within the context of a community of adults and children.

Raddery receives its referrals from local authority education and/or Social Work Departments (as Social Services Departments are called in Scotland). The school charges fees, agreed with the Convention of Scottish Local Authorities (COSLA), and these are paid by the referring authorities. The largest single number come from the authority in which the school is situated, namely Highland Region, and the second largest number come from the neighbouring Grampian Region. A minority come from further afield.

The second part of the book looks at the implications for educational and child-care policy and practice. For example, it examines the justification for this kind of special provision at a time when the role of special schools is being questioned in the light of the growing emphasis on integrating children with special needs into mainstream schools. Are the needs of the children who attend Raddery very different from others who have been successfully retained within normal classes? If Raddery, and schools like it, have a particular contribution, what is the secret? Can it be shared with ordinary schools?

Raddery is not just a school. It offers residential care. The two aspects of care and education are combined in the concept of a residential community. This, too, raises questions in the light of current policy favouring care in the normal community.

In Britain, admitting a child to a children's home is nowadays usually regarded as temporary leading to return to family at home with social work support or as preparation for fostering or adoption. But this policy has not affected the continued demand for some residential communities for children with special needs. Perhaps the two approaches are not inconsistent provided, as at Raddery, links are maintained with the child's parents or other carers.

The notion of community care in the health field as well as in the social services has meant that children (as well as adults) are no longer expected to live in long-stay institutions. For example, children who traditionally stayed in hospitals for long-term care or for other social reasons are now expected to be cared for elsewhere. Old policies and practices are now questioned. But where, in these circumstances, does the responsibility for care lie? The answer is that sometimes it falls to residential special schools to care for children who, in the past, might have been either in children's homes or other special care establishments or in hospital wards.

Successful community care policies require adequate resources, especially adequate staffing. This is true for the integration of children with special needs into mainstream schools. But what kind of resources are we talking about in the case of the children we have described as having 'very special needs'? Different considerations apply here than for children with physical disabilities. Raddery children could be said to have had social disabilities. The emotional damage and the suffering they have experienced are visible in their behaviour. Many, especially the girls, have been sexually abused — a fact which might not have been disclosed a decade ago. Many have suffered from inconsistency from parents or other carers. Many have also suffered from inappropriate responses from the social services and in earlier schooling. In other words, their problems are the responsibility of society as a whole. If they are not tackled, wounds will be carried unattended into adulthood with often disastrous consequences which will affect society as a whole.

While Raddery has no shortage of referrals, some other special schools for children with emotional difficulties have recently closed in Scotland. Was this because some referring local authorities rushed into a policy of 'integration' without counting the social cost? This is one of the questions I will try to examine.

This is not to claim that a school like Raddery can take on 'any child', whatever the problems or whatever the situation, and expect to be able to cope. For some children, Raddery will not be the best placement — at least not at any given time. It is hard to define these limitations because they depend on the situation at the school and the needs of other children. Raddery, as we have said, is a community and any newcomer will affect the life of the community. An aggressive frightened child might at

one stage cause too much disruption without finding any opportunity to learn — and it that case no-one will benefit. In some
circumstances it is felt that if the child had come sooner, more
could have been offered.

The writing of this book was commissioned by Raddery
Council and was occasioned by the school's tenth anniversary
celebrations. It is intended for various groups of readers. First,
and most obviously, it is intended for those associated with
special education for similar groups of children. This includes
teachers, carers, managers and parents. Secondly, it is intended
for teachers in ordinary schools. Thirdly, it is intended for residential social workers and other care staff as well as health care
staff and specialists concerned with emotionally damaged children. Finally, the book is intended for managers and policy-
makers in the agencies which impinge on the children and their
families, including education, child guidance, social work, mental health services and juvenile justice.

I have written this book from several perspectives. For the
past twenty years I have been engaged in social research. I have
been especially concerned with evaluating facilities and services.
This includes finding out what service-users think. In looking at
Raddery, it was natural for me to ask what the children experienced and also to ask parents, as well as those who referred the
children to Raddery for their views.

As a piece of research, what I have attempted represents a
'case study'. There is a discipline in this approach. It involves
describing and analyzing my experiences in ways which place
them in a wider context so that they help to illuminate the
experience of other schools and other residential establishments.

I believe that to do justice to this approach, one has to be
sympathetic to the 'case'. Since Raddery started a little over ten
years ago, I have been closely involved as a member of the
school's governing body, called a Council. I am currently its
Chairman. I have, therefore, a sympathetic interest to declare in
the school I have researched.

I have a deeper personal interest to declare. As a young
man, out of university, I had the privilege to work for a short
time with a pioneer in special education in Britain, namely
David Wills. He had a great influence not only on the lives of

the children and their families but on the future lives of his staff. He wrote many books describing early pioneering experiments which are eminently readable. Amongst other things, I owe to him an example of writing about subjects which could be seen as technical and professional in a very human way. One of the first schools he described for 'maladjusted children' (as they were then called) was founded by him, also in Scotland, called The Barns Experiment, which started in Peebles in 1940. (It later closed to be replaced by other more advanced educational experiment.

Like David Wills, I believe it is possible to write informatively and with integrity from a position of personal involvement. The sort of language I believe he would have approved of would be to say that a school like Raddery is based on understanding and on love. The staff need to understand the children they are working with and to love them. Education is the product. Of course, I am not as involved as David Wills was when he wrote about Barns. He founded and ran Barns. But David Wills also wrote about a famous 'approved' school, Cotswold, when it was in the process of change which eventually led to its becoming a well known therapeutic community, the Cotswold Community.

I, too, am writing about a school that has changed and is changing. But in this case, both the founding of the school and its development are associated with another 'David', David Dean, OBE. The changes are less dramatic than those which affected the Cotswold School which became the Cotswold Community. The changes that have taken place at Raddery could be called a subtle evolution of ideas and practice together with a natural growth in numbers, from some twenty children to the present forty (and a decision not to increase numbers any further.)

If I had written about Raddery during its first few years, it would very much have appeared as a portrait of its founders, David and Valery Dean. It is a tribute to David that this is now less the case. His is still the central and abiding influence. But the descriptions 'facilitator', 'focalizer' (to use a Raddery expression) as well as Principal, would more aptly describe his current roles than 'charismatic leader' (an expression which was often on people's lips a few years ago). This is not to suggest that David

Dean has lost any of his charisma. Instead, the charisma has become the charisma of the school in which staff, and ultimately the children, can share.

I write as someone caught up in this charisma. Yet, more than any of the children, staff or parents, I am an outsider looking in. I have looked 'in' very closely. I have interviewed each one of the staff, some of them more than once. I have focused on a random selection of the children over a period of about two years. Several of these have left and I have followed them through to see what the outcome has been since they left. I have also seen the parents. In addition, I have attended, watched and contributed to, innumerable meetings, activities and happenings in the school, and at a house a few miles from the main school known as Strathallan. Situated in the small town of Fortrose, Strathallan offers a more intimate environment for older children preparing to live 'inter-dependently' (a term which I prefer to 'independently') in the community. Some of these children are now attending the local secondary school from their intensively supported base.

In one respect, my involvement with Raddery is related to some earlier research. In the late 1970s, with Margaret Thomson, I conducted a survey of the needs and services of ALL children in the Highlands and Western Isles of Scotland who were living away from parents.* A disturbing finding was that children who were emotionally damaged were then being sent hundreds of miles away to special schools in Dumfries and Galloway because there was no provision nearer home. David Dean arrived in the Highlands to look for an area where a new school was needed just at this time. The Highland Regional Council were happy to support him and offered premises which appeared very suitable, at least as a starting-point. The buildings have grown and developed — that is one aspect of the story of Raddery which has to be placed alongside the development of staff, of ideas and, perhaps no less important, of public relations.

From both of my perspectives on the school — as researcher and as Chairman of Council — I have no hesitation in saying

---

* SEED, P. and THOMSON, M. (1978) *All Kinds of Care*, Edinburgh, Scottish Academic Press.

that Raddery is a 'very special school' centred on the needs of its children with 'very special needs'. The central question I have set myself to address is what can be learnt from the Raddery experience?

I have been helped in all sorts of ways — far too numerous to attempt to list — by David and Valery Dean and all of the staff and others associated with the school. As an example, this is manifest in the illustrations undertaken by Christopher Fry, at the time a member of staff (since pursuing further education for teaching art).

Everything that is written and illustrated is authentic but, at the discretion of the children, Christian names only have been used in their case. The faces drawn in the illustrations do not identify any of the Raddery children.

Part I

The Raddery Experience

The ambience of the meeting house, David Dean lights candles while children listen to music.

Chapter 2

Raddery as a Community

Morning Meeting

Morning Meeting takes place in a converted loft over the out-buildings of the original Raddery House. An external wooden staircase has been built on to give direct and exclusive access from outside to a warm, carpeted room beneath the beams. Comfortable chairs line the walls to secure the spaces for children and staff to sit as they please. They enter quietly, their individual after-breakfast jobs and 'inspection' (to see that their jobs are done and that they are tidy) accomplished. Candles are lit. Some of the children and adults have been outside feeding animals or milking goats. All have at least walked outside from the main building. Stereo music plays. It is the sound track from the film *Local Hero* — stirring and wild at times but also reflective. More and more they come. The spaces around the wall are filled. More come. A child moves up closer to his neighbour to make space for a new entrant. The next child sits on the floor against a specially made floor-cushion. A visiting adult enters. Immediately a child moves from his secured seat and settles on the floor. The visitor enters the space made vacant. And so the room is filled — with children and adults and filled with stirring music and, at the same time, a sense of quietness.

David Dean leaves his seat, walks across the carpet to turn off the record player beside the door and returns to his place. As he walks, he seems large beneath the low ceiling. He settles and looks for a moment at a fidgetting child, glances at another in recognition of something personal between them and begins to speak.

He talks about his childhood love of Westerns and the experience of the Saturday morning movies. Then he shares the memory of being a child himself amongst a group of children who went for an expedition. Times were harder in post-war Britain than they are today, he explains. People were poorer. Just going on an expedition was exciting. But later, he tells the Meeting, he organized trips himself. One trip, for example, had been to Iceland. He asks how many children have been abroad. A surprising number raise their hands. He talks with the children bringing them into the conversation and leads by stages to breaking the news that, following his visit to Russia some weeks ago, a special school in Leningrad had invited children and staff from Raddery to visit their school. In return, it was planned a group from the Russian school would spend some time at Raddery. The news is given by the children (whom he had prepared) in dramatic form by their reading the correspondence with the Russian school.

Each member of the Meeting has books of hymns and songs called *Alleluja*. When the news is broken, David asks everyone to sing *Strangest Dream*. Then he goes on to discuss some of the practical implications of the visits. The numbers first suggested by the Russians would have to be reduced. Their school was much larger — for 200 boys. He turns to Eric — Eric Carbarns, the Assistant Principal Family Care — and asks if he is a betting man and, what odds he would place on the visit taking place? Eric replies 'It is a cert'. Will Eric choose a hymn? The pace of the Meeting is slowing and Eric choses *Blowin' in the Wind*. By the end, there is a complete stillness. One by one the children begin to leave interspersed with staff as the record from *Local Hero* is re-started with the invigorating song *Three-Way Flier*. There is no set order. A child from one side of the room meets with another at the door. The candles are extinguished. Nearly an hour has been spent in Morning Meeting before classes begin.

Each Morning Meeting is memorable. David Dean normally takes it twice a week. Bill Badger, the Depute Principal, takes it once a week and other senior staff take it once a week. Staff are drawn from a wider group to take the Meeting on the fifth day in the week.

Here is my record of another Meeting taken by Bill some months later.

A record was playing lively love tunes by Buddy Holly. Bill then told us something about Buddy Holly and how famous he was in the 1950s. He went on to generalize about famous people and good people. He gave as an example Nelson Mandela. He asked the children what had happened to Mandela recently. One replied: 'He has gone home to be with his wife'. 'Yes', said Bill, and he wondered what it must be like after over twenty-seven years in prison to be free? Through question and answer Bill told the Meeting how yesterday Mandela had persuaded previously warring tribes to throw their weapons into the sea. What power Mandela had! Bill said 'Mandela had not always been like this. In his early days he had not been particularly good to his family and had left his first wife'.

Bill went on to mention other well-known people and then he distributed pieces of paper and pencils to each Member of the Meeting — children and adults. He asked each of us to write down the name of a person who would be known to others and who was powerful and good. While we thought about it we were asked to sing (unaccompanied), what appears to be one of the favourites in the book — *Blowin' in the Wind*! When we had finished, Bill said that the song summed up many of the things we had been talking about.

The pieces of paper were collected and Bill selected one from the middle of the pile. He explained that he was going to ask us to try to guess firstly who had chosen the name on the paper and, secondly, why. The name was Steve Biko, the African nationalist who had been killed, or died falling, after police interrogation. A member of staff was correctly guessed and he owned up that he had recently been reading Biko's biography.

Another random selection from the pile of papers produced 'The Queen'. It took some time to trace the
choice to one of the youngest children, Yvonne, though
others, including a member of staff, had chosen her too.
Why 'The Queen'? It proved demanding for Yvonne
to try and explain, with help from her staff 'team-mate'
sitting next to her offering to prompt. 'Because she
travels', Yvonne said. 'Had she seen The Queen?' 'Yes,
when she visited Elgin'. Was she beautiful? 'Yes, she is
liked by people'.

The next choice was 'God', chosen also by more than one
child. Questions open to all the children produced their
profile of God. He was the Person who made us. Without Him we wouldn't be here. He died for our sins. I
reflected that no child seemed able quite to say that God
loved them. The school does not preach 'religion' but this
was an example of a religious discussion coming naturally
from the children in a way which had meaning in their
lives.

Unfortunately there was no time for any more. Names of other
choices were read out: Mother Theresa; Gorbachov; John
Lennon; George Bush; and so on.

What a feast it had been! No two mornings are identical.
Sometimes, for example, there is dancing or activity involving
physical touch.

This particular Morning Meeting had been without four
children who had absconded. This was a serious incident, but
Morning Meeting was not the time to consider it. After classes,
it was taken up in a subsequent Community Meeting, which
Bill Badger also took because David Dean was attending a
Council Meeting (the school's governing body). I was sitting
next to David at lunch when he caught up with the news given
to him by other children at the table. The four boys, I learnt
(who had since returned) had been a great nuisance the night
before. Only one of them had been able to face up to the
seriousness of his behaviour. But Bill seemed well pleased with
the meeting with the children, which had been long and had

made them all late for lunch — a matter which concerned David because food carefully prepared was on the table. At the end of the meal, David, who chaired the meal, apologized to the kitchen staff that a lot of people had been late. He said he understood that on this occasion it was for an important reason but that he didn't like it to happen often.

As a therapeutic community, Raddery has many different kinds of meetings for different purposes. The daily Morning Meeting is the centre-piece. It invokes healing at the deepest levels of each child's experience. It is the heart of the deliberately created caring environment. There is structure but very little set form — in other words, you never know quite what to expect. It starts shortly after 9.00 am when children and adults make their way individually and take up their seats. There is always music and always a quiet time. The main part is set by the adult taking Meeting who chooses his or her own way to draw upon the best that there is from within the adults and children attending.

It is difficult to analyze the full process of the Meeting. In terms of complex social interaction, it would take many pages to describe one Meeting! In a more general sense, and with an element of mystery, it is about the whole approach for which the school stands — addressing the spiritual wisdom which is to be found in each one present. It is a harmonic foundation for the healing and educational work that is to be accomplished that day.

I asked David Dean to explain to me the origins of the particular form of Morning Meeting at Raddery. He answered my question with stories of his past experiences on the staff of a school where you were expected to talk to children for a week about a set topic, for example 'Love'. He found he could not do it.

I didn't have any confidence that I had anything to say. I wasn't one of these people who could stand up and talk about love for a week. You had to be clever to do that and I wasn't clever. But I was good at encouraging children to be participants rather than just an impassive recipient of my wisdom.

So, as he put it, he had to think of 'other ways':

> I wanted a room which didn't confuse issues. I didn't
> want to take a room which was ten minutes' later used
> for table tennis or maths or something. I wanted one
> room, with the right colour and texture and lighting,
> which was set aside for creative spirituality or whatever
> you want to call it.

And in the first school where he was headmaster, Cartref Melys
special School, in North Wales, David found a hay-loft for this
purpose. 'The staff were really puzzled', he said. 'I remember
having to work quite hard to keep the space because they would
have loved to have filled it with other things for the rest of the
day'.

Apart from the hay-loft in North Wales, the lay-out of the
Raddery Meeting Room owes much to a room called the Sanctuary at the Findhorn Foundation Community near Forres. The
Sanctuary is a circle of chairs in an ordinary building where
people enter either individually or, as a group, for what is called
'atunement'. David explained he did not want to put fancy
words to it, so 'We call it a quiet time which is absolutely
pitched at Raddery's level'.

The form of the Meeting also owes much to Abbotsholme
School, where David was English master and Head of outdoor
education, when the headmaster was Robin Hodgkin, a well-
known Member of the Society of Friends (Quakers). A Quaker
Silence is not passive but is the way actively to find, as the foun-
der of the movement, George Fox put it in the seventeenth
century, 'That of God' in each of us.

> I wanted — on the Abbotsholme model — lots of people
> to share in the talking. I didn't want to monopolize it
> and I wanted people to agree to a fairly common format.
> For instance, music at the beginning and a quiet time at
> the end and, in the middle, that's up to you and your
> creativity.

The spirit of Morning Meeting was not always easy for new members of staff to understand, especially if they had come from a conventional school. David Dean explained:

> It is an amazing way to start the day because it is unprovocative. What do you normally start with in a school? (If you start with anything now.) When I was in school it was a hymn, the Lord's Prayer and then a monologue from the Deputy about the graffiti on the loo walls. In other words, a confusion of words which just made you want to get out.

The Morning Meeting has to be powerful. It has to be worth taking nearly an hour of 'prime time'. So what was so valuable about it, I asked? David answered promptly:

> Well, it's bonding. It's the bonding of the community and it comes after — you have to put it in context — children going off, possibly alone, doing their morning responsibilities.

So Morning Meeting fulfils a personal commitment to the value of each child and a corporate commitment to the School as a caring community.

Yet to some children as disturbed as those at Raddery, even the word 'God', preached by an adult, could have meanings far removed from the Love of Jesus. So, even after a silence at the end of a meal, David prefers a form of Grace which simply says: 'For food, we give thanks'. David feels, moreover, that any specific religious commitment could be divisive and detract from the willing expression of spirituality within the school community as a whole.

At Raddery, the spiritual door is always an open door. Morning Meeting, the Grace after meals, and, hopefully, everything that the staff convey by their own beliefs in daily action, keeps that door open.

I have started an account of Raddery as a community by a lengthy description of the spiritual dimension, partly because people often find it hard to think in these terms when it comes to special education. We can talk easily about smaller classes, one-to-one or small group counselling, shared responsibilities, meal-times — even about a holistic approach — but how is spirituality expressed as the embodiment of wholeness? Well, the answer I have described requires a lot of experience and a lot of history.

Staff Support

Another cornerstone in Raddery's community is staff support, captured very well in the last HM Inspectors Report.* In summarizing the then thirty-eight (now forty-four) staff, and their wide range of qualifications and background, it states:

> The aims of the school include the creation of a community which is not affected by considerations of qualifications or status and to which all can contribute.

This could easily be misunderstood. A superficial understanding could suggest it to mean that staff qualifications do not matter in a therapeutic community. The reverse is the truth. Qualifications, taken in the broadest sense to mean appropriate formal courses of training and a wide background of experience coupled with right attitudes and motivation matter even more at Raddery than in a school which might not aspire to be a therapeutic community.

Each year, the school produces a staff list detailing each member's function and background. Let us, by this means, introduce some of the staff for the year 1989–90:

Greville William Badger (Bill). Resident Depute Principal ...

Bill, it was, who took the Morning Meeting described earlier. He is the Deputy Principal ('Depute' in Scotland), which means

---

* SCOTTISH EDUCATION DEPARTMENT, SCOTTISH OFFICE. HM Inspectors of Schools. *Raddery School, Fortrose. Report of an Inspection in May/June 1986.*

he has to manage the school in David's absence. He has responsibility for much of the running of the school in any case. 'Resident' means that he lives, with his family, in one of the school's houses — in his case on the periphery of the estate.

> ... MA, Oxford University, Psychology and Philosophy; Postgraduate Cert. Ed., St Luke's College, Exeter; Dip. Ed. Psychology, Birmingham University, M.Phil, Lancaster University ...

By any standards, Bill is well qualified academically as a teacher and as an educational psychologist. His experience matches this:

> ... Educational psychologist, Handsworth, Birmingham; Head of Middle School, Moorclose School, Workington; formerly Head of Experimental Special Unit, Wyndham School, Egremont, Cumberland.

When I interviewed Bill for the book, he told me: 'I tend to be at the sticky end of kids'. That statement must ring true for many a school deputy! Behaviour problems which get out of hand in class or during an out of school activity tend to get referred to him. But where Bill's position differs from that of a deputy in a school with a conventional hierarchy, is that Bill expects, and is expected, to play his part, as an equal member of the community at a deeper level where each person's contribution is valued and supported, whatever it is, alongside the contribution of all the other staff. Mutual support is not just a nice idea or a slogan. At Raddery it is a necessity. Bill, for example, is not the best administrator in the school — quite a deficiency in a conventional deputy head! He himself needs a lot of support, not only from David but from some of his colleagues in carrying out his responsibilities. In turn, he gives a lot of support to others.

One of those who is good at administration is Eric. Before Bill was appointed, Eric served briefly as Acting Depute.

> **Eric Carbarns**. Non-Resident Assistant Principal (Family Work). BA Econ. (Hons. Soc. Admin), Manchester

University; MSc (Social Studies) and CQSW, London
School of Economics ...

Apart from having a degree, Eric is a qualified social worker
with many years' social work experience in two Scottish local
authorities. Unlike Bill, he lives with his family in Dingwall,
some fourteen miles away from the school. Rather less than half
of the staff live within the school area, partly because of lack of
space and partly because it is regarded as a good thing that while
some staff live within the Raddery community, others are part
of the community outside. Many live in nearby Fortrose or in
the nearest village called Rosemarkie.

Eric's post ensures that an appropriate level of contact is
maintained with families. He arranges reviews and gets to know
prospective children and their parents. But he also has responsibilities within the school. The fact that he lives fourteen miles
away — and that he has duties with the families — does not
absolve him from evening duties and week-end duties with the
children or from playing his part in informal educational activities in the school.

Eric is the first to admit that residential work with children
— for example, being on duty when children are going to bed
— is not what he is best at. His experience is in field social
work, as it is called, and he has had to adjust. In a slightly
off-guarded moment, he told me: 'The school has sucked me in'.
(Again, I am sure social workers at other residential schools will
understand just what Eric means!) But he recognizes the necessity for this. His regret is that there is not enough time to do all
he would like with families. The link between residential social
work and 'field social work' is a necessity in a school like
Raddery for two main reasons. The first is in order that the
child's problems at home can be understood in the light of their
behaviour at school, and *vice versa*. The second is to support the
parents through the adjustments that they have to make when
their child first comes to the school and as he or she develops.
But to do his residential job, Eric needs a lot of active support
from his colleagues.

Alf Smith, Resident Team Leader, was one of the earlier

members of staff to be appointed soon after the school opened in 1979.

> Resident team leader (Teacher/Houseparent). Cert. Education. University of Birmingham. Formerly taught mathematics and science and housemaster at Ncholenge Secondary School Zambia, Kanjuri Secondary School, Kenya and Borbora Secondary School, Uganda.

Alf is respected as perhaps the person amongst the staff who can above all be relied upon to give support at the deeper level of community involvement, beyond his formal roles and duties — important though these are. 'All my previous jobs', he told me, 'involved boarding schools'. This, he feels, has helped him to look into reasons why particular behaviour occurs at Raddery — amongst children and sometimes amongst staff. In answer to my question about what had changed at Raddery since he came, and what the community had learnt, he said:

> The philosophy remains the same. Staff have to find it and the philosophy is self-perpetuating. It is a philosophy of caring and understanding the child's behaviour but at the same time accepting it and still liking the child. If children know we like them they don't mind taking a telling-off.

At the time when Alf said this, he also felt, in common with others who had been at the school since its early days, that it had lost something of the meaning of community as it had become larger. It is fair to say that a lot of work has been shared within the community during the past year to understand these feelings and look at the many factors concerning both staff and children that contributed to them.

The children now being referred are more disturbed and damaged and need greater intensity of care than did most of the first children who came to the school ten years ago. I will look at the reasons for this later (see Chapter 6). But this has led to greater demands on staff and increased a sense of frustration, especially when some children cannot cope with even limited school holiday periods without intensive support. These sorts of issues have meant that the community has needed to become more complex — and this is, perhaps, fundamentally the more important problem than the numbers of children and staff (although it is recognized that forty children should be about the maximum for Raddery).

The Community Becomes More Complex

The first 'complexity' to be introduced to the Raddery community was the opening of a 'half-way' house in October 1983. It is an ordinary, large old house, called Strathallan on the outskirts of the small town of Fortrose, about three miles from the school. Its purposes have changed. This was one of the things that concerned Alf when I talked with him:

> Originally it was to take older children as a half-way house but, because of troublesome children who had caused an embarrassment in the village, it has changed. Now there are some children aged 14 at Strathallan but older children aged 16 at the main school.

This was shortly before the series of discussions both at Strathallan and with the whole community I have referred to.

It is useful to mention at this point where the School Council and its members fit into the community. Raddery is formally governed, as a limited Company, by its managers who form the Council (elected annually from a larger group of Members or 'Friends' as they are termed). In practice, they were initially the people David and Valery Dean gathered around them to start the school. Thus, the idea of the school, which was the idea of its founders, pre-dated the formation of its management committee. Membership has changed as the management needs of the school have changed. For example, there are now more members with a professional educational or social work background compared with a financial or legal background or with buildings expertise, than there were in the earlier days — though the Council tries to maintain a balance in this respect.

Gradually Council members have become incorporated in policy and development decision-making alongside school staff rather than in a traditional management style where the Principal was regarded as the appointee to be accountable (along with the school's firm of accountants who act as bursar) for everything that happened.

The use of Strathallan was one such issue where Council members became involved. The problem was that Strathallan was being used for a range of different purposes and reasons which were not always compatible, but which basically reflected the more complex needs of children now attending the school. A group was appointed in August 1989 comprising two Council Members, David Dean, Eric Carbarns and two of the Strathallan staff, Martin McDonnell and Stuart Bates.

I will continue the process of introducing some of the staff as we go along:

Martin McDonnell. Non-Resident Assistant Principal Half-Way House. BA (Hons) Geography (London); MA (Hons) Anthropology (Auckland, New Zealand). Post-graduate Cert. Ed. Special Needs, Geography (Lancaster). Formerly Head of Humanities at Selly Oak School, Birmingham.

Stuart Bates. Non-resident Assistant Half-Way House. BSc. Civil Engineering. (NE London Polytechnic). Formerly in agriculture and forestry.

Strathallan staff have duties within the main school as well as at Strathallan. For example, Stuart has duties in the school workshop and also teaches keyboard instruments.

The Council Members attending the group that met in the comfortable and relaxed Strathallan sitting room were Dick Poor, a retired Director of Social Work with long child-care experience, and myself. Dick began by asking a lot of questions about Strathallan. The house had been originally staffed by David and Valery Dean and then by another married couple. Next, it had been led by Elizabeth Spence — a long-serving member of staff who had had posts in the main school as houseparent and then team leader before coming to Strathallan for three years. She had recently left to go into the Ministry of the Church of Scotland and Martin had taken over.

Dick Poor wanted to know exactly when Strathallan was open and when it was shut. The answer was complicated in detail but, roughly, Strathallan was open for half of the total vacation periods of fourteen weeks in the year, together with term time. In other words, it was closed for seven weeks, including for two of the six weeks of the summer break.

Martin and Stuart described the situations of children using Strathallan during these holidays periods. Mostly, they concerned the prospect of breakdown during holidays otherwise spent at home and they were a very different group from the normal term-time residents. The latter attended as part of an organized programme for school-leaving or, in some cases recently, as preparation for staged integration into the local Secondary School — known in Scotland as the 'Academy'.

David pointed out that the Strathallan staff had been appointed to provide preparation for independent living whereas the children needing holiday care or 'respite' were mainly those who had not been at Raddery long and who needed continuing care, some even on a fifty-two-week basis.

The meeting moved towards discussing how the Raddery community as a whole could respond to changing needs. I noticed that David was keeping silent so I asked him how he responded to various possibilities I could envisage. He said he was listening. The discussion went on for a while and then David said he had an idea. He lay on the sitting-room carpet and drew a diagram (see below) depicting a two-way relationship between Strathallan and the main school and also between the school and a new unit he envisaged to take mainly younger or 'newer' children who needed continuing care. These ideas were welcomed and we began to discuss the implications for staffing, for funding, for buildings and so on.

CONTINUING ⟷ MAIN SCHOOL ⟷ STRATHALLAN
CARE UNIT   ↘   ↙
                              OUTREACH

David Dean's Diagram at Strathallan Meeting

Discussions around these themes continued over the next few months in various forums involving the school's professional consultants and in staff groups. In particular, a key role was played by Pat MacGoveran, a local clinical psychologist; Colin Keenan, a social work lecturer from Robert Gordon's Institute of Technology at Aberdeen; and the most recent new consultant, Melvyn Rose of the Peper Harow Foundation in London. Earlier, the local Director of Social Work for the Highland Region of Scotland, Jim Dick, was also consulted. Some of his staff had been concerned about the care of a particular child at a time when Strathallan was closed.

In the following Spring (1990), consultants, staff and Council Members met for their annual conference which, this year, was on *The Future of Raddery*. One of the questions was whether, as Raddery had become larger, it should in some way be split up. Apart from the pressures on Strathallan, there had been pressures in the main school. Some children clearly needed more close and individualized attention. Others needed protection. Some specialization seemed to be needed. But the community needed to hold together. David Dean felt he did not want completely separate 'houses'.

There were more staff working-parties and more meetings.

The answer that came up was based on the idea of 'venues'. These are separate locations for specific living requirements. But the extent of separation is flexible and controlled.

Five such 'venues' were identified:

1 *Strathallan* — now to revert to its original purpose as a half-way house, and also to develop the outreach work the staff were keen to undertake.

2 *The Cottage* This comprised two staff cottages, which were to be joined together to form a living unit for 'five of our least integrated children' — as David described it to the Council. The precise definition of the term 'least integrated' reflected the experience of another special school, the Cotswold Community in England with which Raddery had developed links (see Chapter 5).

David later explained the approach to the Council as follows:

> Children in the cottage can be part of the full programme of the community only if they are able to manage. If they are withdrawn from the programme — because the cottage is staffed at all times of the day and night — it is possible to be positive about their alternative programme. In the cottage garden is a new departure for Raddery and that is the establishment of a Foundation area. Several cottage children are time-tabled for one-to-one work in Foundation.

The idea of a 'Foundation Unit' was borrowed from another special school, Peper Harow.

3 *Harris* This 'venue' resulted from a splitting up of the living accommodation in the main building into three areas. Harris was described as being for six children who were 'quite vulnerable':

> They are also young and the domestic refurbishment of Harris has allowed an atmosphere of security and attractiveness to pervade.

4 *Skye* Another part of the main building was to be for two remaining girls — normally there would be more girls in the main school but it happened that over the previous year several had left and boys had come in their place.

5 The remainder of the *Main House* for boys who, as David later put it in a meeting with parents, 'are on the move'.

Children at each of the 'venues' have breakfast and tea separately, but, on certain days, lunch together at the main school. This arrangement makes for more individualized attention and regains a sense of intimacy within each 'venue' which some staff felt had been lost as the school become larger, and which, in any case, was now necessary to meet the needs of specific children.

All these changes were finally agreed in July 1990. They were to be implemented for the start of the new school year

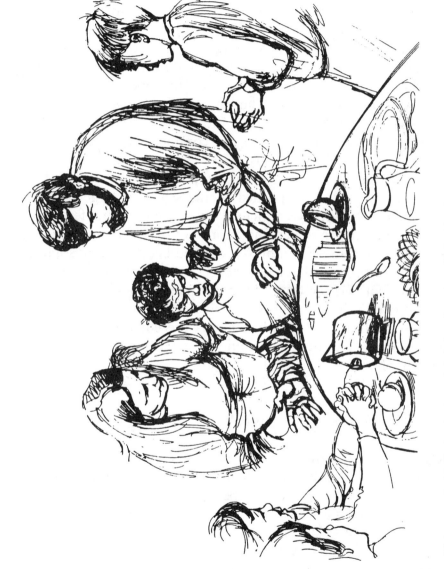

Dining room incident, showing two adults in tune & coping with the situation.

in September — only weeks away! There were immediate implications for alterations to buildings. A hectic building programme, using mainly the school's own staff for carrying out the work, was undertaken during the summer break.

There were also major changes in the deployment of staff and, indeed, in some staff roles. 'Teams' of staff and children were to be based on each 'venue'. But to bring a sense of wholeness around what was going on in the school community — and in practical terms to ensure co-ordination — a senior member of staff was to serve as 'daily enveloper' for a complete twenty-four-hour period. The details of this were still being discussed and worked out during the school's 'community week' when staff meet alone before the commencement of the new school year.

So, to get back to Alf's original point he made to me about a year before all this happened — the school is larger and less cosy after its first ten years than it was during the first few years. The community has become more complex because children have presented more complex needs and because more sophisticated and more professional responses have been called for.

Incidentally, the other point Alf made about children causing trouble in the village is something which only rarely occurs. The establishment of Strathallan was preceded by involvement of the village community including meetings in the town and at the school.

Professional Teamwork

Raddery as a community has gained in confidence and become more ambitious. Elizabeth identified some of the key parts to this in an interview shortly before she left. Strathallan had provided what she called 'a new dimension with adolescents'. The creation of Eric's post in family work with an emphasis on the idea of treatment with families and the coming of Bill to be Depute, with his emphasis on professional skills and assessments, had been important milestones. One could add that the increased involvement of consultants from psychology, social work, child psychiatry, organizational analysis, as well as special education, has helped to sustain these ambitions and build on confidence and the potential for professional teamwork.

Professional teamwork within the community of Raddery is structured around teams (staff and children), team-leaders and others who are called 'envelopers'. The 'envelopers' comprise the team leaders, together with other key senior staff.

In describing the role of the 'envelopers' to me, David Dean compared the notion with the more common idea of a 'core group' of staff which, he said, was a concept used in Steiner communities. Long-standing members of a community hold the focus of commitment to the ideas of that community. 'But', said David, 'I wanted to find the antithesis of core group, especially something opposite to hierarchy' and, in discussion with another member of staff, David Tidmarsh, the idea of 'enveloper' was conceived:

> The envelopers form a notional circle of strength into which every other worker can step knowing that they are being supported by the group.

For example, 'envelopers' are expected to 'provide a secure enough framework for new workers to get their feet off the ground'.

I found that David Dean could not explain the 'envelopers' without discussing his own role and his determination to try to resist an exclusive charismatic leadership which, he feels, unless it is resisted, 'disempowers' other people. Perhaps the idea of 'envelopers' is a means of sharing such a leadership without the disempowerment of others.

Such an idea carries high expectation and David does not hesitate, when necessary, to express his disappointment. 'One of the problems we have at the moment', he said when I interviewed him in the summer of 1990, 'is that there's actually as much strength outside the enveloper group as there is inside it. It's something I made something of in our meeting the other day and I was quite honest'.

I had, as it happened, been talking with some of the 'envelopers' shortly after their meeting with David and he was not underestimating the impact of what he had told them. Occasionally — perhaps not too often — just because staff members of a community have learnt to accept one another, they can accept, as children can, what Alf called 'a ticking off'.

Both David Dean, and the staff concerned, did something about what was, in effect, a near crisis of confidence in the 'envelopers' at that time. For some, it confirmed that the moment had come for them to think about moving on from the school — not because they were in any way inadequate in carrying out their formal responsibilities — but because they lacked the informal authority which is essential in leadership in a non-hierarchical community structure.

Part of David Dean's response was to re-cast a new post in the form of Assistant Principal (Care) which would attract the kind of person to achieve the strengthening the community required and, at the same time, address the underlying situation which gave rise to the crisis. This was the increased strain on all of the staff, as the school responded in the more sophisticated professional ways I have described earlier, to the increasingly complex needs of the children.

A developing, professional community entails tough decision-making in tough times. But at Raddery it is not a case of decisions being made FOR people (except perhaps in only one or two extremely unfortunate situations I can think of in its first ten years). Staff (or 'workers' as David prefers to call them) are — as distinct from children whom they work for — 'adults' and, as adults they are expected to take adult decisions for themselves. But the context is one comprising both intensive support and confrontation with others, guided by what they see as the truth. Indeed, one could say that support and truthful confrontation are two sides of the same coin in a therapeutic community. But if truth is interpreted exclusively by the leadership FOR the others, not only are the others disempowered as David rightly perceives, but the community — as many experiences world-wide have testified — is doomed. It is a delicate balance, but one which, in my judgment, Raddery is achieving.

Team Work and 'Ethos'

Professional team work in any residential establishment is partly sustained by the sharing of ideas and the development of what is sometimes described as 'ethos'. The ethos of Raddery is very strong and it is constantly sustained and developed. One of the major opportunities for this is the annual staff conference held at the school for a full week — the week before the children return after the summer break. All the staff attend. Much of the task is specific preparation for the coming term and the coming year — assimilation of new arrangements, new timetables, new allocations of staff duties. Part of the time is spent in the staff teams discussing the assessment and treatment plans for individual children. The staff also meet together as a whole — and part of the time they play together.

The headings for some of the sessions for the conference this year (1990) illustrate the underlying awareness of sustaining the ethos for effective teamwork:

Planning for the one-to-one's (children and staff); Individual/group therapy; Team mate time; Social, educational, cognitive assessment, — the flesh on the bones.

The role of the daily 'enveloper'.

Talking our way through a day.

Maintaining standards and efficiency under new arrangements.

How do we improve our child progress/planning — giving the children 'a way ahead'?

Packed lunches and an afternoon of staff/people centred activity (e.g. barbecue/picnic, a game of rounders, groups going off far and wide to activities of their choice).

Team Work with Children

I mentioned earlier that the idea of 'envelopers' had been jointly conceived with another 'David' (there are several in the school!), David Tidmarsh. It is time he was introduced:

David Tidmarsh. Non-resident Team Leader. Teacher/ Houseparent. Cert. Ed. Charlotte Mason College, Cumbria. Formerly of Outward Bound School, Locheil and Shotton Hall (special school), Shropshire.

I had the privilege of attending one of David Tidmarsh's team meetings, and to give the flavour of how one such meeting operates, the following is part of my account:

> I arrived to find David T's meeting in progress and a child immediately put a chair in place for me at a table to sit down. A major item for consideration was one of the children who was being teased and it was explained by a staff member that this hurt him particularly because of its meaning in terms of home circumstances. During informal conversation with the children it was discovered who had been doing the teasing.
>
> The meeting shaped responses in terms of shared policy towards each child.
>
> A point of general interest to me was the use of thumbs up or down to express approval or disapproval of the performance or behaviour of particular children. It was possible to put one thumb up and one thumb down or one thumb level and one down and David T., who acted as chairperson, counted thumbs up or down in each case to give the information to the child. This was a very effective visible sign of group pressure on the child.

Perhaps an underlying sign of the extent to which a community is therapeutic or not is the extent to which negative sub-cultures are absent. I say 'sub-cultures' in the plural because in a formal hierarchical institution there is likely to be both a negative sub-culture of children, inmates, patients — or whoever the objects of the organization's existence supposedly are — against authority and, at the same time, a parallel sub-culture or cultures amongst the more junior staff. I would not claim from my observations that either is entirely lacking at Raddery — or perhaps in any therapeutic community — but it is minimal on the staff side and kept within quite tight bounds on the children's side. A team meeting is one example of how Raddery is structured as a community to bring into the open the kinds of events and feelings affecting the lives of children, and sometimes adults, in a controlled way where they can be handled constructively.

'Events and feelings' are not always as civilized as they appeared at David Tidmarsh's meeting on the day when I attended. There have been other occasions, when I was gathering material for this book, when staff were physically assaulted, children absconded, children sexually assaulted other children, and so on. This must be expected. The school would be either failing in its task or redundant if it were not so. But these things do not happen unknown or unseen by others. Nor are they left unanswered or not fully dealt with, or swept under any carpets. Most of such events, and much else that forms the life of Raddery as a community, apart from being dealt with instantly, come before the main weekly community meeting. This comprises all the children and a large number of the staff (i.e. the staff who are available to attend or who need to attend).

Shared Responsibility with Children

The team meetings and the Community Meeting provide a structure where children can, amongst other things, share with staff (or 'workers') the responsibility for the running of the school insofar as this is helpful and consistent with the healing process.

Children (and parents) are aware that children come to Raddery to learn in an environment where they will experience this healing. But Raddery, as a healing and a learning environment, is what the children, as well as the staff, help to create. Recognizing this is the core of what is meant by a therapeutic community. Children are a resource, not just objects at the receiving end. They will help to heal others. Sometimes, it is true, especially in the early stages, they will help only to lead others astray or contribute to other's (and their own) suffering.

But as these situations are dealt with, with staff and children working together, a new experience through a new dominant culture is generated.

One sees that for this to be successful, everything that has been said about the community in terms of staff support, leadership and shared values is essential. Yet 'troubles' are kept in context. Community life is about living, with all of its 'colours of day'. The format of the weekly community meeting reflects these colours.

Community meetings begin and end with short periods of silence. The agenda structure is based on the notion of 'temperature readings' developed by an American therapist the late Virginia Satir. As adapted for Raddery, these include 'items of information', 'minutes', 'complaints' or 'problems', 'expectations', 'appreciations', and 'what I want for myself'. This last, namely 'what I want for myself' is a particular feature of the smaller and more intimate community meetings at Strathallan. The Raddery Community meetings held at the school are larger and more formal, with all of the staff and children attending, including the children from Strathallan. David or, in his absence, Bill chairs the meetings but a child keeps the minutes. 'I suppose', David told me, 'the community meeting is showing that we are not averse to looking at the dirty linen side. It's there. It's best to put in on the table and acknowledge it'. Early in the agenda are 'action points' from the last meeting, followed by 'problems'. Children are asked to put their problems in writing 'rather than have a whole flotilla of half problems and no problems masking the real ones'.

David pointed out to me that not all staff — and not all children — feel comfortable at first contributing in these large meetings. But even if they do not speak up or speak out they still play a part as what David called 'witnesses', especially in relation to 'appreciations'.

> When the appreciations come the children are as much
> involved even if they have not been involved in some
> of the other stuff. You can get group euphoria in appre-
> ciations and in these instances, especially when a boy
> who has consistently lied about his actions for years

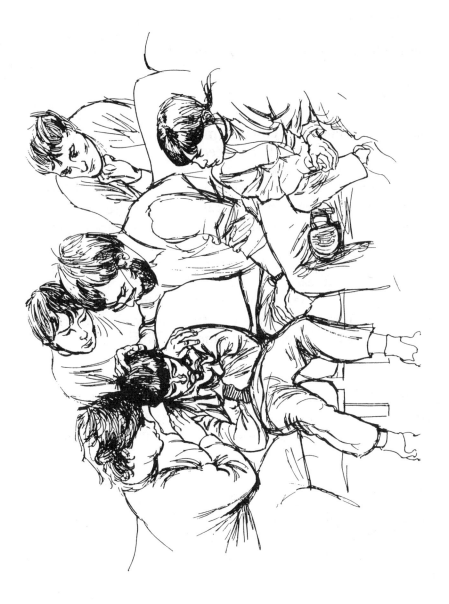

An uncomfortable moment during community meeting.

and years — the fact that he can be witnessed saying 'Yes, I did it. I pinched the other boy's radio and I smashed it'. — and then getting applauded, not for his actions but for the stage he had moved to in being able to say 'Yes, it was me'. Everybody gains from that. It's not just the boy who made the move but everybody who was witness to it.

'Appreciations' come towards the end of the agenda. Earlier on there is many an uncomfortable moment for a child faced with the combined pressure of staff and peers.

However, the pressure is in the context of support. I remember when I was a child at a boarding school the head-master would use silence as a means of pressure to try to discover the perpetrator of a crime. I remember it because, even though I was not the culprit, I would blush on the culprit's behalf with my own discomfort. The procedure at Raddery is designed to make it easy, not hard, for children to come to terms with the consequences of their behaviour and often this means there is not undue pressure to identify the culprit in public. My notes of one community meeting illustrate this:

Bill was in the Chair. David B. was appointed to keep the minutes in the absence of the secretary. Bill explained that there were no major items today and most of the time was spent on a large number of complaints. Amongst these were the following.

A number of children had been teasing and tormenting animals. Four children were named. In discussion, Alison (a child) made the good point that none of these children would do it by themselves but that they did this when they got together. Animals, it was agreed, were very important to Raddery. There was then a vote on two motions — one suggesting a ban on contact with the animals and the other a ban plus compensation. The latter was approved and the children were given some mucky jobs to do.

Gerry reported that his hammer had been taken from the workshop even while they were working. It was known that some children had been involved including Lee and Danny. The hammer had been broken. An issue was made about how important the hammer had been in the past. (Lee was not at the Meeting). No-one was going to own up to this but a number of speeches were made stressing that compensation should be made in this case as for the misdemeanours towards the animals.

Alison's bicycle lights had been stolen. They had been purchased with money borrowed from Jenny (worker) and they were expensive. She was still paying the money back. Again, the procedure adopted was to bring out how important the lights were to Alison and the children were encouraged to speak their mind about what they felt. It was not known who had done this and no-one was going to own up. It was agreed that the school's lights, which are kept to lend, should be given to Alison meantime and it was pointed out that other children would not have the school lights. In this way, the whole school was making reparation.

William's trousers had been torn. Again no-one was going to own up. Again, it was stressed how important this was to William because they had been given to him by his mother. During the process William was reduced to tears and another boy got up and sat next to him to comfort him.

There was a review of the School's Fun Day efforts ... One activity was 'muck throwing' (at people) ... The total raised was £78.67. Bill Badger pointed out that the amount was not the important point. The main person who had done most for the muck-throwing was Lee (who had also been in trouble on other items).

To summarize, the main regular meetings which are the framework for the operation of the therapeutic community at Raddery:

MORNING MEETING — Daily. Staff and all children.

COMMUNITY MEETING — Weekly. All staff and all children.

TEAM MEETING (or VENUES MEETING) — Weekly. Staff and children in each venue.

STAFF TEAM MEETING — Staff meeting separately in each team.

STAFF MEETING. Weekly. All staff.

ENVELOPERS MEETINGS. Weekly. Envelopers.

CLASSES MEETING. Twice each week-day. Children and staff in each class.

TEACHERS MEETING. At least once a term.

PARENTS MEETING. At Annual FAMILIES GATHERING.

COUNCIL MEETING (School's governing body elected from ANNUAL GENERAL MEETING) and its FINANCE AND GENERAL PURPOSES COMMITTEE. three to four times a year each.

Other groups include SHARED RESPONSIBILITY GROUPS, ACTIVITY GROUPS, and STRATHALLAN groups — and I am sure there are others I have left out!

As David Dean recently said, Raddery has become a complex organization!

David and Valery Dean

David and Valery Dean are the co-founders of Raddery. The community derives its special features and characteristics from their shared vision. David is the school's Principal. Valery has currently several roles. She is a part-time remedial teacher. She is the 'focalizer' (a Raddery term) for animal keeping. She plays host with David to many visitors. She has a relationship with the wives of other members of staff who live in the Raddery community. With David, she attends Council Meetings.

David and Valery met when they were both on the staff of Abbotsholme School. David was an English master and Head of

Outdoor Education. Valery was Head of the Geography Department and an assistant housemistress.

I interviewed David and Valery separately, and at leisure for as much of a day as was needed, at my own home to try to understand better their roles in relation to Raddery. The relationship between them exemplifies the mutual staff support on which the community depends. They do not always agree. As David put it:

> I can't resist saying to Valery on Friday when we get home eventually, 'What was it like in community meeting?' For that matter, 'What was it like in staff meeting?' I suppose it's a bit of wanting to know that I'm still doing what I ought to be doing. Also, and she's very good at this. She doesn't play back what she thinks I want to hear. She plays it straight back and it's a very useful sounding board to me.

From Valery came the corresponding comments:

> We share the vision of the same ideas and developing things. We talk together, particularly in the holidays. I have stayed in tune with David over the years and have known where Raddery was moving from and to.

Valery described her role in relation to David as 'quite easy' — and that is very much the impression the other members of the community and visitors would have. They appear utterly natural together, as colleagues and at the same time as family within a larger family community. The two aspects of their partnership run together. As Valery explained:

> I am a working wife. We live in a working home — an extension of David's own room. He comes home and works by telephone. And he communicates with a number of people from within the school once he gets home.

What then, is the shared vision that holds together David and Valery and the charisma of Raddery?

Like everything worthwhile, with a spiritual foundation, it is love. I asked David, was it not that emotionally damaged children were entitled to nothing less than the best? He replied it was part of the theme of Raddery in its 'caring creative environment'. And he continued:

> It's not only the best. There is a good reason for that, and that is the business of compensation for previously omitted childhood experiences in terms of tactile development and bonding and warming and all the rest of it. It's very difficult to compensate for that but I see no alternative but to go overboard in creating that environment. The critic who comes along and says: 'Ah, this child's home isn't like this so what's the reality of this?' And you say. 'Well, that's the whole point, the fact that the child's home never approached anything like this is why they are here in the first place. And the community response to that, plus the sort of individualizing of their identity and fostering — that is exactly what the place is about'.

Later in the interview he added a couple of further points. 'First, you tended', he said, 'to over-compensate, quite legitimately, sensory opportunism in making sure you don't miss a trick. You get every possible advantage from your physical provison, from your mixed staffing, from the way you use the day, and I think mood setting is incredibly important in the therapeutic community'.

Finally, David added, in commenting on an experience where the children had shared for one evening the castle Great Hall, with the music and fire burning in the grate, belonging to the then Chairman of the School Council, Lady Cromartie:

> It was all nurturing in a way that simply echoed what we were trying to do for our children. This is back to the charismatic notion about the school because you can't do these things if you are hidebound by rules and regulations and that's part of the message, part of the holistic approach.

Chapter 3

Raddery as a School

Raddery as a school must be understood in the context of Raddery as a community. Raddery aims to be a caring, educational and therapeutic community comprising adults and children.

The Holistic Approach to Education

'Holistic' has dimensions — one could say it has length, breadth and depth. The 'length' dimension is that each moment of each day can be educational for the child (and, incidentally, often for the adult). Mealtimes are a good example of this. Bed-times are another. Then there are the kinds of domestic activities like animal-keeping that children engage in, especially in the early morning immediately before Morning Meeting. (I will return to animal-keeping as an example a little later).

'Holistic' education has breadth insofar as it embraces every kind of endeavour to engage every facet of the child's life and potential in the educational process. In terms of broad activities, this incorporates at Raddery everything from summer camps, hobbies like cycling and canoeing, to visits abroad — most recently for some of the children to Russia. It tries to take account of the full range of moods, colours, sound, movement, shapes, textures. It offers physical and emotional care, as well as intellectual stimulation and development. It provides protection, sometimes through rules — for example Raddery's no-smoking rule.

Take Lee's encouragement to have mud slung at him to raise money, described earlier when it came up at a community meeting (see Chapter 2, page 37). It is impossible to draw a line here between recreation, education and therapy. The educational aspects included the physical coping with unpleasant sensations and being tough enough to receive physical discomfort in a socially acceptable context. They included the social acceptance of being the butt in fun from his peers and from staff. Wider aspects included developing a sense of awareness of social concerns in the world outside for which money was being raised by Lee's efforts and which he was instrumental in helping to organize. At a therapeutic level, all of this was a new and contrasting experience for Lee, as Lee the Good, when so often — even in the same Community Meeting — he seems to be Lee the Bad. The release of the goodness opens the door to education, as, therapeutically, it opens the door to acceptance of the 'bad' in a context of the understanding, exploration and development of Lee the Whole Person.

Holistic education has depth in that it involves the whole person of each staff member engaging in the whole person of each child. So far I have used my own words to interpret what I think Raddery believes in so far as holistic education is concerned, but let me now quote David Dean. He was telling me about a discussion amongst staff:

> The staff were attempting to define holistic in our school the other day for themselves — well, no, not for themselves, for the school — and they didn't get further than saying it was the education of the whole child. They were so busy talking I didn't get a chance to say anything ... I will later!

> Holistic for me means that it's not multi-disciplinary. It's a whole concept beyond multi-disciplinary. It's where — yes, of course the worker brings their skills, but not only do they bring their skills — they allow part of what they are as human beings to be shared with the children in a very real way.

David went on to explain the application of this to staff appointments and staff involvement:

> The way it comes through is that if you are appointing a cook you are also also appointing her as a sister or a grandmother or whatever her personal role in life is. I am expecting some of those qualities to come through so that she works in a grandmotherly way or a big sisterly way or another way — knowing full well that that's dangerous because it's with these figures that the children have had most difficulty.

In contrast, the teacher who reserves and preserves their role is more protected because the teacher is, by and large, the person with whom the child is not angry, David said. He cited some examples of what this could mean for the un-protected, risk-taking staff member. One elderly member of staff had been kicked by a little boy and she was off work for three weeks with a swollen leg. David explained how this involved the whole school:

> Part of us felt enraged and desperately protective of her and sad and furious with the child. Yet we had to hold all that because we knew that this child had been contained in a drawer by a grandmother. The staff member represented part of that for that child — far more than me. I mean I wasn't going to get kicked. I might have been in another context. I'm far more likely to be assaulted by a boy who had a very rough time with his previous head teacher. And yet I have more skills to protect myself against that sort of assault and I could contain it better than someone who is sixty-four.

If we have highlighted the risk-taking in being so personally exposed, many of the experiences of staff involvement with children, using every moment for educational advantage, are mutually rewarding. For example, as in other residential establishments, children like to gravitate towards the kitchen and, while this has to be controlled in the interests of getting the work done, the educational opportunities to be derived from children helping in the kitchen are not missed.

From this point of view, however, David emphasized that especially because of the wide age-range of Raddery children, one must keep in balance the needs of children also to be 'cared for'. Contrasting Raddery with another therapeutic community school where there is an older group of children, David explained:

> When you are dealing with children at the age of 10, 11 and 12, there is a positive caring, nurturing role to be undertaken by the staff and you can't abdicate that in favour of some well, We must do it all together. Children can contribute ... but they musn't feel responsible for it.

Even at Strathallan, the half-way house, there is a danger that education could become too extensive at the expense of caring.

> Children are supposed to cook, budget, prepare, wash up, sort the house. Okay, but they also have to go to school, to have work experience, and you have to say at one point: 'Wait a minute, we must get the balance right here'.

So at Strathallan, there is one part-time domestic staff member. At the main school, apart from the cooks, there are a number of local 'houseworkers' who are expected to combine their functional role with the educational and caring roles I have described.

Food at Raddery — what people eat — is important. As Isobel, the cook, explained:

> We tend to talk about well-balanced good food rather than wholefood. The problem is getting children to adjust to it. Perhaps nowadays more of the families are doing fast foods at home — eating out of tins. Sometimes when a new boy comes he will hardly eat for a week and then he gets used to it.

> Some children have diets. For example, one child cannot take red colouring in food and this affects the cheese —

we changed to colourless cheese. Other children, for example, cannot take lentils. One child cannot take tomatoes.

At Strathallan there is greater emphasis on educating children to make choices about food. A sheet in *The Strathallan Handbook*, produced for the children, reads:

MUNCHIES
YOU DECIDE WHAT WE EAT

Menus are made up for about two weeks at a time. Lunch is always a light meal because people will be off on work experience.

Tea is our main meal of the day. You should make sure we eat a balanced diet.

Chocolate cake and ice-cream every night is NOT balanced!

The adults will help you with this at the beginning but soon it will be an easy task.

You will also have to make up the shopping list for the BIG SHOP! Pay attention to items that are SUGAR FREE and REDUCED FAT etc.

If it's a choice between brown or white, brown wins every time!

FOOD GLORIOUS FOOD

At the level of individual contacts between staff members and children, formal counselling merges into day-by-day informal educational contacts between staff and children. These, again, are both educational and nurturing. David reported to me what Bill Badger had said when they had discussed this at one of their regular weekly meetings:

We were talking about one-to-one counselling and how it needed to be a cornerstone for next year's programme.

And we agreed that counselling wasn't just sitting down, you here and me there, and away we go. It was the nudge in the corner. It was the raised eyebrow across the room to ask to modify what they were doing. It was saying 'Oh, that's nice'. It was the moving on. It was so many levels of connection.

Education then, is fundamentally about 'connecting' with children all of the day, in school and out of school. And at Raddery, this means connecting with children for whom personal relationships have fairly consistently failed to make connections in the past.

Classes

Let us now turn to the more formal aspects of schooling. Each class is different, reflecting the personalities of the teachers and the different needs of the children attending. But whatever the differences of style and content of class teaching, the attempt is made to address all of the needs of the whole child in class, as out of class.

Classes comprise about five to six children. Classes are not numbered but named according to the Christian name of the teacher. This happens informally at many ordinary schools. At Raddery it is also official practice.

Here are brief descriptions of three contrasting classes I sat in on.

First, I sat in one day on David's English class — not David Dean, but another David, David Tidmarsh whom we introduced earlier in connection with the idea of 'envelopers' (see page 29, Chapter 2). Five children were attending and I sat between two of them, Margaret and Michael, around a hexagonal table. I noted that David was spending an unequal amount of time with different children and, by chance, most of it was with my two immediate companions. Michael, aged 13, was doing an exercise where he had to write answers to questions about a piece of text which was in the form of a newspaper report of a train accident. He was asked to read it aloud — not

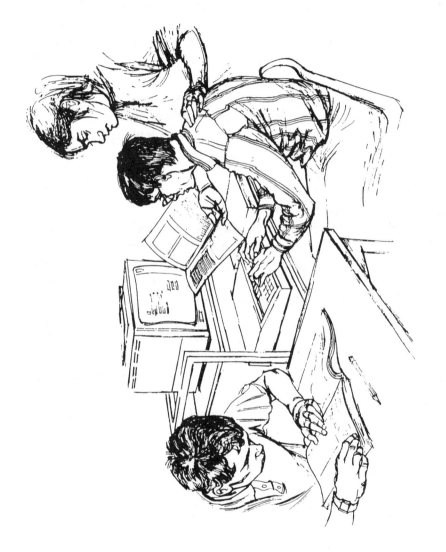

Supported learning in the classroom.

for the whole class because the others were getting on with their own work, but loud enough for David and also myself to hear. Then the answers he had previously written down on paper were praised. 'But they could be improved' added David. For example, he had repeatedly used the word 'it' in several answers as a lazy way of avoiding saying who or what 'it' was — for example, 'Was "it" the train driver?' Well, how about writing the "train driver" then?' Michael squirmed slightly but did not seem unhappy.

Meanwhile Margaret, aged 13, on my other side, seemed to be finding it hard to stay awake. When David moved on to talk to her he told her that he would be more lenient toward her today than he might otherwise have been because she had been very energetic in connection with the Fun Day — the one where Lee, described earlier, had had mud slung at him. Margaret had been on a sponsored run to raise money.

Margaret was supposed to be doing an exercise similar to Michael's. In her case, the newspaper story concerned the habits of a hermit crab. Margaret did not appear to be impressed. She sloped across the table. Bill Badger entered the room with a message and, at that point, Margaret began to cry.

I was aware that Raddery expects its visitors to participate appropriately — depending on who they are and how well they are known to the children. I did know Margaret a little, so I tried to indicate some interest. David encouraged me to do more in response to Margaret's crying. I became a little more involved with the story and with Margaret, as I would have done with one of my own children having difficulties with homework. But soon David came to give her the attention she was craving. She leaned against him, quite large and heavy though she is, like a baby but he rejected her continued wish for cuddles, saying this was not the time nor the place and he gently tried to coax her to do her class work.

Moving round the table, the next child to Margaret was Colin. He took quite a long time to settle but then worked quite well. At one point he threw a rubber across the table towards Margaret which I happened to catch. David told me afterwards he had deliberately not taken this up in class but had spoken to him during the break about it. (I didn't go into the reasons for this). Next to Colin was David K. He was immersed in his bookwork and neither wanted, nor received, much attention. David Tidmarsh told me afterwards that he rushed on ahead and then, when he found he had made mistakes, he would be upset. At one point he had got up to get himself another book to read and David Tidmarsh had stopped him.

Secondly — and over a year later — I sat in on part of David Reid's class, also for English, but, as he explained, heavily influenced by Standard Grade requirements as well as 'SCOTVEC' for options in (1) social and vocational skills; and (2) planning an expedition and executing it.

Five children were sitting round a table with David discussing the translation of a story (reproduced on a sheet each had in front of them) by Guy de Maupassant. It was the story of a trawler that sailed into a storm. The waters had calmed sufficiently for the skipper to decide to risk putting the net down. His younger brother, amongst the ship's small crew, got his arm caught between the cable and the ship's side. The drama was about the skipper's decision not to cut the cable to free him because the net and the potential catch of fish were too valuable. The younger brother's arm was cut to pieces.

David was careful to let the children give the answers to questions he posed about the dilemma faced both by the skipper and by the crew carrying out his orders. He gave minimal steerage to the conversation to broaden it.

The attention span seemed fairly good, but there was also a behavioural agenda. This was to do with children not interrupting or, as David put it, 'cutting across' each other. At one point, there was a digression because some of the children were throwing salt crystals (from a previous class) at one another. David stopped the class discussion to deal with this, using the same group approach i.e. a discussion of the issues. After a few minutes, the discussion returned to the de Maupassant story.

The children were responding in very different ways. David afterwards explained that (before I had come in) the discussion had been chaired by a child but he had felt he had had to take it over. It seemed to me there was a leadership issue in the group. One of the children was the leader in the task agenda concerning the story. He was engrossed in it and was not interested in the behavioural agenda. Another child was interested in the story, but also in the salt-throwing. A third was only minimally concerned with the story. There were, indeed, a lot of interruptions for David to deal with and he dealt with the two kinds of interruptions — the verbal and the salt throwing — in a unified way of encouraging recognition of the advantages of allowing people to be heard.

At the end, David asked the children what they thought about discussing stories like the de Maupassant one. A concensus reply appeared to be that they preferred discussing the 'real' stories in the news, like the Gulf crisis.

A sixth child, who had been absent during most of the time re-appeared at the end. He had been asked earlier to take his jacket off and when he did not want to do this David had given him the choice of keeping it on and leaving the classroom or staying with it off. He was welcomed back and politely asked to do some extra work to catch up. Apart from a little haggle over when he should do it, it was readily accepted.

The third class I attended was 'Jenny's class'. This was a younger group. The theme was colours as part of science. They were following a project work card. The atmosphere was very informal. Children scattered to a work place of their choice (desk, table, widow-sill, floor) to make drawings with crayons. As they completed their tasks, they returned to Jenny who was standing beside a small projector into which different coloured slides were inserted. As the drawings were filtered through the different lights, the children could see some of the effects on their drawings. Some parts were missing when the drawings were projected onto the classroom wall. One child was especially excited to see the wheels of a car missing. Another intelligently caught onto the potential for this exercise and came back with a sequence of drawings in different colours making it possible to demonstrate a pilot being ejected from his plane. Meanwhile another child had drawn a person. When Jenny asked who it was he replied 'Pat MacGoveran' (the consultant psychologist). There was then laughter all round as the green light showed him with his trousers missing. The child went away to add other features to the picture — a house and his car. I noticed that Jenny did not follow up discussions about what pictures might mean, but focused on the topic which the class was about — namely the effects of the different colours.

The children were enjoying the drawing and the class gradually wound itself up with the enthusiasm which Jenny engendered. When some children became bored with the exercise towards the end of the class, they were allowed to make coloured decorations for Christmas.

A behavioural agenda during this class arose when children had difficulty sharing the crayons. One child went into a sulk because another would not lend him a crayon. Jenny quite easily talked him out of it by suggesting that this was not the most effective way to get what he wanted.

At the end of class, there was an incident when one child switched on a personal radio. This was allowed but another child tried to take the connecting cable off him. This boy said he wanted to take the cable home to give to his father and Jenny explained that it wasn't his and that he couldn't take home anything he liked to give to his father.

What conclusions can we draw from these three examples of the content and process of class-room teaching?

First, behaviour is managed through discussion rather than by overt control and, secondly, such discussion is integrated with the educational purposes of the class, within a structured curriculum. Each class has educational and therapeutic agendas, but they are not, as far as possible, dealt with separately. A holistic approach can be seen to try to hold together all that the child needs in a given moment of time — wherever and whenever that moment is — in this case in a class and within a structured concept of learning. This does not mean that every need the child presents will be dealt with on his or her terms. Margaret was denied a cuddle. A child was not allowed to wear his jacket in class. A child was not allowed to take away part of a radio. But each child's demands were recognized by the adult and, perhaps, thereby acceptance was conveyed of a kind the children had not readily experienced in their previous schools.

The experiences of each class are continued, and brought together, in what are called 'daily meetings'. There are two such meetings, one at the finish of morning classes and one at the end of the more informal activities at the end of each afternoon.

David Dean chaired the meeting I attended after I had been at David Tidmarsh's and Jenny Gray's classes.

There was a contrast here with the classes I had seen in the way behaviour was controlled. David Dean was very strict in stopping the proceedings to ask, or politely but firmly demand, that children stopped fidgetting. He explained to the meeting that time was short to cover all that the meeting had to get through and that they could not afford to be interrupted or not listened to. He also dealt there and then with children who were not wearing 'school clothes'. (Raddery does not have uniform, as such, but there are certain rules about clothing allowed at particular times).

David seldom lets anything slip by when he chairs a meeting, but he dealt with these issues very speedily to concentrate on the business, which mainly comprised reports back from each class. Teachers and children contributed. The items reported included both educational and behavioural issues, though behavioural issues tended to come to the fore in discussion. But the quality of work, for example, of the children in Jenny's class in making the coloured decorations was praised. David Reid's class report was partly in terms of the efficiency of the work done but there was discussion about one of the children who, before I had arrived, had lapsed into swearing. The fact that there was so much discussion was because it concerned a child who had a particular and long-standing problem with swearing.

Throughout the discussions David Dean was skilfully referring to the topical interest in the Prime Minister, John Major's school report which was on the news that morning. It had not been a particularly good report either in behavioural terms or educational attainment.

During a lift back to the station that day, I talked to David Dean about the educational programme. He emphasized the educational component of afternoon and evening activities as well as the morning classes. He thought that they would be concentrating more on pre-vocational objectives where many of the children had strengths for example, he said they would do 'brilliantly' in the SCOTVEC modules on social and vocational skills and on leading an expedition. So far as standard grades were concerned, he thought they should be mainly concentrating on English and on arithmetic.

The educational objectives and methods of the school were formally reviewed by HM Inspectors in 1986 (see page 18, Chapter 2):

> There are six classes, consecutive by age ... Three ... follow a modified primary school programme, two work to a secondary school-type of organization and the sixth follows a course which emphasizes work experience and preparation for independent living ...

> In the secondary classes the main emphasis in the formal curriculum is on specialist teaching in English, mathematics and science supplemented by experience of art, swimming, sports, practical skills, outdoor education and a variety of other activities, some taught formally, others very informally in keeping with the ethos of the school ...

> The school operates a three-term year with three half-term breaks ... The school day starts with the Morning Meeting at 9.10 am and ends with a short class meeting at 4.45 pm to review the day's proceedings; there are substantial breaks at mid-morning, mid-afternoon and lunch-time.

The Inspectors might have considered the conventional word 'break' something of a euphemism in view of the hub-bub, for example, of important happenings in the mid-morning break when staff and children — and often visitors, such as prospective parents, social workers, psychologists or Council Members — are milling about in the same room! We have referred earlier to the educational importance of meal-times when, also, much school therapeutic and educational business may be conducted. But 'breaks' do describe a change from activities, in the mornings at least, conducted for most of the children in something resembling a 'class' in the sense that they are usually sitting down and 'working' with the assistance of a 'teacher'.

To continue with the Inspector's Report:

> Teaching methods and styles are appropriately informal and pupils generally respond well ... Much of the work, particularly in English and mathematics, is based on individual assignments and individual support. The scope for pupil choice is limited by constraints of timetabling and resources, but staff have excellent detailed knowledge of their pupils which can be put to good use and in planning activities and allocating roles ...

> Teachers generally keep brief records of work undertaken, pupil progress and topics to be covered, and pupil performance is reported at staff/pupil meetings, mainly in behavioural terms. In the secondary classes, and in relation to outdoor education programmes, a more systematic approach to assessing and recording pupil mastery of learning objectives has been adopted ...

There have been some changes at Raddery since the Inspectors' visit in 1986 and especially since the review of Raddery undertaken in 1990.

First, a new Foundation Unit has been established adjacent to the Cottage (see page 26, Chapter 2). The term 'Foundation Unit' is borrowed from another school, Peper Harow. Children are attended to on a individual basis or in very small groups. Activities include therapeutic play — the first thing I noticed when I visited the unit shortly after it had opened was a very large Lego set, and a child playing with it. There is also a soft play area and a messy area is being developed. There are sometimes trips out. The Unit is mainly for children who would be described as not integrated enough to benefit sufficiently from their class-work without this additional style of educational input and attention, much of it on a one-to-one basis. The furnishing and *milieu* of the unit is one of intimacy and secure warmth. There is a sofa and easy chairs, for example. The school's psychological consultant, Pat McGoveran is closely involved in the work of the Unit.

Secondly, classes are no longer (if they ever were) strictly 'consecutive by age' as the Inspectors stated. Social compatibility and the stage the child has reached will be taken into account. There is flexibility in choosing the class from which the child will most benefit, taking everything into account including other children's needs.

So far as records are concerned, teachers do now keep records of educational attainments as well as statements of intent.

Like all schools, Raddery is influenced by national developments in education. In Scotland there is no 'National Curriculum' as in England, but the equivalent is a series of working papers on *Curriculum and Assessment in Scotland — A Policy for the 1990s* for which the school is preparing. Meanwhile, the needs arising from the new Standard Grades system have been addressed. Spencer Houston, the Assistant Principal (Programme) at Raddery, told me that relatively few children would benefit from the Standard Grades programme. Like David Dean, he said he would favour more emphasis on SCOTVEC. This is a broader system of entry to vocational courses and qualifications than the English National Vocational Qualifications (NVQ). It is a modular learning system and, Spencer told me, creates less anxieties than the traditional system of taking a group of formal examinations at the same time.

The general differentiation between morning and afternoon activities has been maintained. Spencer told me the emphasis for most morning school activities was what he called 'provision' of basic education, whereas the afternoon placed more emphasis on 'experiential' learning. Some houseparents are involved in teaching in the afternoons. Music was an example he quoted — 'musical experiences to touch the soul'.

'Animal-keeping' is an interesting example of an 'outdoor education programme' with a 'systematic approach'. Three members of staff are involved and (for the year 1989–90) seven children. A document produced by the group sets out:

1   Skills objectives
2   Therapeutic opportunities available
3   Individuals involved and the areas seen to be potentially most useful to them at this stage.

Under the first heading, 'skills objectives', separate lists appear for goat keeping, sheep keeping, and for hen, duck and geese keeping. For example, for hens, ducks and geese:

1 Safe housing at night
2 Feeding and protection
3 Collecting and storing eggs
4 Recording egg production
5 Bedding down, mucking out
6 Care of midden
7 Care and maintenance of tools and equipment
8 Economics of poultry rearing
9 Rearing of young birds

One must remember that Raddery is in a rural area and that many of the children come from rural backgrounds so that some, at least, of the issues raised will have an already familiar context.

The second, 'therapeutic opportunities available', is very broad. To quote just three out of 11 sub-groups:

A. Experiences of job simulation, *viz*: application, apprenticeship, negotiations and notice-serving in resignation; opportunity for promotion to Head Keeper by election on the basis of performance, experience and leadership; liability to demotion from job on grounds of performance, reliability or other.

C. The chance to have instilled reasonable levels of economic awareness through avoiding wastefulness and aiming towards self-sufficiency in care of animals.

G. The experiences of team working and group interaction, as these affect the individual and the efficiency and harmony of the working whole. This may involve mutual support of a practical or more personal nature, problem solving on either level, with or without adult support, and may call upon high levels of resourcefulness, commitment and integrity.

The other sub-groups of therapeutic opportunities, not quoted in full, cover:

> Challenge to develop personal organization
> Opportunity for hard physical work
> Responsibility through trust
> Opportunity for group decision-making
> The chance to be with animals
> Sharing the life experiences of animals
> Challenge of leadership

Under the third heading of the animal-keeping document, the relevant parts under the first two headings are identified to make up the individualized programme of activities and learning for each participating child. For example, for William, who was looking after ducks, most of the skills were devoted to many of the therapeutic opportunities listed.

When I interviewed Valery Dean, one of whose special duties was with the animal-keepers programme, she told me of particular past children who had specifically benefited. For example, one child wouldn't communicate at all for several weeks. She couldn't even eat a meal with others. She couldn't even enter a room when others were present. But, after a while, she opened up in talking with a goat she was looking after. After this, she began to talk to others in school situations.

Another child had sadistic tendencies and used to crunch up small animals in his hands. Valery said it was a risk putting him in charge of animals, but it had worked. As he was given responsibility he became protective towards animals.

Yet another child, aged 15, had been very depressed. She had thought there was not much for her to live for. But as she became attached to a particular goat that was not thriving, and she nursed and minded it, 'her thinking improved'. She began to feel happier.

Of course, no one activity can be taken in isolation from a total educational and therapeutic programme for each child. The above examples show how just one of very many activities specifically helped.

Reintegration with a Local School

It is possible for a child to move on from Raddery to attend a local school during the day-time. I followed the discussions concerning this possibility for a particular child, Zoe. It began at a teacher's meeting I attended late in 1988.

Alf described previous attempts with earlier children attending a local primary school. It had not, at this time (1988), happened at the Academy. Initial plans were made for the careful preparation that would be required both at Raddery and at the Academy. It was agreed 'we can only go so far at this meeting without Zoe herself being present'. One of the teachers, Suzie, made the point that Zoe could be demanding in class but perhaps she chose to demand in a special class setting more than she might in a normal class. Alf made the point that if we waited for the time to be perfect for the move, it would not take place until she had left Raddery. David Tidmarsh said children came to Raddery to take time out of normal schooling and that they might not achieve their full educational potential until much later. Bill Badger said it was worse to try and fail than not to try.

In discussing the history of Raddery's attitude to integration more generally, it was suggested that the question had come up at secondary level at this time because there had been an emphasis on work experience recently and this had helped to develop thinking towards the idea of integration in school. Work experience had increased because of a group of children who were practically rather than academically oriented and who were therefore more suitable for work experience. There had not been, they said, any lack of belief in the principle of integration. But now Zoe, who had academic ability, raised the issue of integration in the school more generally.

Zoe's future schooling was raised at various other meetings during the following four months including a staff meeting I attended at Strathallan. By this time, it had been agreed that Zoe would be attending the Academy for English and Maths on an introductory basis prior to full-time attendance during the term following. The item concerned a practical question of whether the days of the year when Strathallan was open would coincide with the Academy's term-time. It was agreed she could stay at Strathallan during all of her term-time periods. After lunch at Strathallan, Zoe was sitting next to me during their small community meeting. When it came to the agenda item 'What I want for myself', and it was Zoe's turn, she said she wanted people to support her if ever she felt weak about going to Fortrose Academy. 'I want people to tell me that I said I was going — if ever I say I don't want to go'.

During the following term I visited Fortrose Academy with a member of Raddery staff and learnt how well both Zoe and another Raddery child had settled in. We were assured that neither staff nor, it seemed, other childen, were at all aware of anything different about the children from Raddery. However, the Academy teachers pointed out that Zoe would have to cope with increased academic work pressures during the following year.

Education with Parents

Education extends outwards from the children to parents. This process can take place through visits, reviews, meetings, David Dean's termly newsletter to parents and at the Annual Families Gathering.

Parents are encouraged to share publicly some of their emotions surrounding their children's achievements as well as their own coping with past problems. Zoe's parents spoke of their experiences to local radio during an annual Families Gathering (1988).

Mother: In my naivety, I think I thought that if I offered Zoe a loving, caring family environment that any difficulties that I certainly saw that she had would all melt away. But the reality is — and it's perhaps something that parents who may feel guilty if they're in the situation where they're not coping well with their children should think about — that love in its own right doesn't actually solve anything. What you

actually need to combine is love and understanding and the ability to have that special way
of managing.

The decision that any parent takes to send
their child away out of the house has actually
got to be painful and very hurtful and if there is
anyone out there who is perhaps in the position
of perhaps feeling they should make the decision, they have really got to grasp the nettle
because it's selfish not to do so.

Father: I think that what has to be said about Raddery
is that it's a place that gives children who have
got tremendous talents — and some of them
have been seen today — but also who have a lot
of problems, a chance to use their talents to overcome those problems.

It also gives parents an opportunity to
recognize all the positive things that their children have, to build on those and hopefully
eradicate the problems.

(*BBC Radio Scotland,*
26th September 1988)

This last point the father made, and similar feelings expressed at
parents' meetings I have attended, show the potential of parents
to learn through participation in their children's learning.

Education and Public Relations

For David Dean, a good image and good public relations are
essential to the educational process at Raddery. Maintaining a
high standard public image and a high profile help to keep an
independent school, especially, going. As a charity, Raddery has
to raise money and agencies referring children have to be able to
see what is going on in ways which do justice to the school. Yet
the children can also benefit directly.

The quality of the image has to be nurtured. A small
example, perhaps, is the high standard lettering the school uses

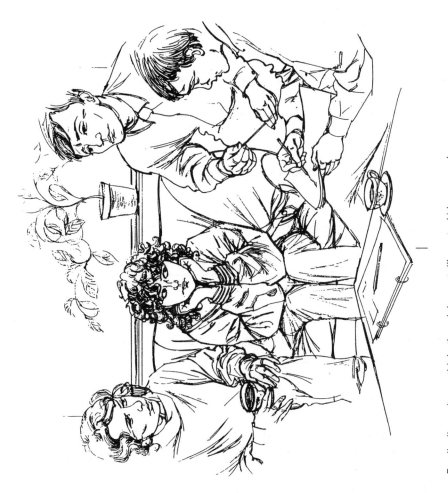

Family discussion — thinks the adolescent: 'I'm not a kid anymore.'

on its notepaper and for its logo. The school transport, like the Raddery pullovers (in a choice of colours) bear only the letter 'R'. Staff may wear them too and I have one myself. The educational component of public relations for the children is around the theme of broadening out, enlarging their lives and helping them to 'make connections' (to use one of David Dean's favourite phrases) between their own lives and experiences in the world outside. Media interest in the school, which is considerable, can be constructive. Why should not children's activities and their contribution to the school's successes be newsworthy? Newspaper cuttings are often sent to parents as well as to Council Members. If the school has such an image, justifiably cultivated, the children's image of themselves may also be enhanced.

Raddery's Educational Approach

What, then, does the educational approach of Raddery add up to? Can one say more than we have already stressed in terms of a holistic approach? Is there anything that distinguishes the educational approach at Raddery from the approach a good learning support teacher would want to adopt in an ordinary school?

When I put these sorts of questions to David Dean, he acknowledged the complexities of the issues and reflected in terms of his own beliefs and the needs of the children.

First, he stressed what he called 'enhancement — a feeling of self-worth that comes from educational achievement'. For most, but not for all, of the children, he regarded formal educational methods as an essential therapeutic tool. A number of strategies, he said, were used. Recognizing that different teachers had different methods of teaching as a 'craft', he spoke of the need for 'combining ingenuity, enlivening and galvanizing'.

He pointed out that the HM Inspectors' Report wanted, on the one hand, more formal curricula activity and, on the other, group therapy. This was 'a tall order' which, nevertheless (as I had witnessed) they were attempting in English. But many children could not sustain the efforts because of 'emotional things going on'.

David said he reacted against Standard Grade examinations. SCOTVEC used continuous assessment which he described as a 'kinder process'. He spoke also of the danger of some too-clever teaching schemes which could deskill the teacher. He kept stressing the teacher's ability to individualize, to respond. The problem was that because every child was so different, children at Raddery were very difficult to group.

Perhaps, the conclusion is that there is not anything special about the formal education, as such, at Raddery. What is special is the context and the opportunity to practice it — small classes, staff support and, fundamentally, its integration into the mainstream community experience which Raddery offers. Specifically, classes follow the morning meetings described at the start of Chapter 2 when the holistic approach to education, as well as to the meaning of community, finds its deepest expression.

Perhaps 'enhancement' is a good word to express a thread that runs through Raddery's educational work, based on holistic principles.

Chapter 4

The Raddery Experience Viewed by Children and Parents

So far, in portraying the Raddery experience, I have largely relied on my own observations and on the views of key staff members. I have only referred to some of the children to illustrate what the school is about, for example in classes or in a community meeting. It is time to bring the children to centre-stage.

This has not been easy. Seldom have emotionally damaged children in residential schools been written about except in terms of illustrating their problems.

I wanted to write with the children, not just write about them. This has had two implications. First, I have had to avoid sensitive areas of past history which children did not want to be published. Secondly, the material has been gathered over a period of about two years, as well as drawing on previous history.

The first step, towards the end of 1988, was to explain to all the children what I wanted to do and why. It was agreed that everyone's name would be put in a hat and that I would select eight names. There was a little 'cheating' (or as a researcher would say, 'structuring') to ensure we had at least one girl and representatives from a range of classes, but essentially it was a random sample of the thirty-nine (at that time) children in the school.

I then talked with each of the selected children briefly and asked them to keep diaries for a week. These were structured, for example, in terms of 'What did you do this morning?' 'Who were you with?' 'Who did you meet?' ' Did anything unusual happen?' And so on.* When the week was over, I spoke with each child about the diaries and what was important to them at Raddery. A further feature of the study was that, for the same week that the diaries were kept, I asked every member of staff for their comments on their encounters with each of the selected children. This gave me a series of portraits from many different perspectives.

Later I visited the parents or other carers of the selected children and, in some cases, spoke also to the agencies which had referred the children to Raddery in the first place.

Eighteen months to two years later I again interviewed the children and most of the parents. I also kept in touch with the children during my visits to the school in the intervening period. The accounts that follow draw on all of this material.

I will begin by comparing two children, Jamie and Paul, who have come from a background of difficulty in ordinary schools and who have clearly benefited from their time at Raddery.

Jamie

Jamie was aged 13 when I first met him and he had been at Raddery for three years. He told me he was previously at different primary schools (which he named) in a small town, some thirty miles away, where his parents lived. He had a younger sister, aged 10, at home with his mother and father. He said the things he liked doing best were milking the goats at Raddery and 'going home'. He told me the names of each of three Raddery goats and how much milk each one gave.

Jamie did not find handwriting particularly easy, but he kept his diary for the full week. From this I learnt school classes included spelling, for example, and French. Amongst many activities there was mention of art, games, kite-flying — 'the kite string snapped' — activities with a micro-computer and 'the

* For details of this approach see SEED, P. (1990) *Introducing Network Analysis in Social Work*, London, Jessica Kingsley.

goats'. An adult was usually mentioned beside each activity and identified with a Christian name — but sometimes other children also featured. For example, he went out to the beach with Kate (staff) and Lachlan (child).

When we come to Friday, Jamie's diary records that he went home and visited his old school. There are no comments. On Saturday, at home, we are told, he 'Stacked 1 ton of logs with mum and dad' — and in the evening watched TV. On Sunday he 'walked the dog' at home and in the afternoon 'came back' (to Raddery).

Staff comments for the same week revealed incidents Jamie had not cared to mention (indeed the diary structure had not been 'incident'-oriented). For example:

An incident in the dining room Tuesday or Wednesday. He made noises after the bell had rung. He was sent to stand up, i.e. by the door. Afterwards, I learnt he was forced into it to some extent and therefore I sat by his bed later and talked to him about it.

And on the positive side, another staff member told me:

Jamie got me to join Amnesty International. He and Richard (staff) are starting a group.

In Jamie's case, indeed, staff tended to divide into those who saw his good side and those who saw mainly his less good side:

My relationship with Jamie involves just the usual banter. I tend to see his good side.

And in contrast:

A wee pest! I try to help him with his language.

Alf recorded:

I occasionally have to say 'Mind your language' and 'Don't be so loud' and then we have a chat.

And from one of the cooks:

> He is around the kitchen quite a bit. He comes in for a chat. I spent quite a lot of time chatting last week. He comes in to see me every day. He is usually moany. He complains about food. I manage to turn his moans around.

Jamie was also attending cookery classes.

Comments from other staff showed Jamie playing a responsible role helping non-swimmers in the swimming pool. Name-calling was a continuing problem however:

> He likes calling me names. In team meeting I brought up that he was continuing to say to me 'You old witch'. He is a good worker in other respects.

In general, then, there is a side to Jamie which is very helpful and which staff are trying to build on, while helping him to see the anti-social aspects to his behaviour. He has problems, too, about his weight and physical health. An earlier medical report I saw said he had been suffering from post-traumatic headaches and occasional dizziness and also that he had an over-sensitivity to noise. At that time (a year earlier) he had also had to avoid heights. But now, it seemed, he could manage scrambling on the sea-coast:

> On Saturday afternoon we went for an expedition along the coast. We were scrambling. This highlighted how unfit he is. He has poor height/weight ratio. He is good at things that require concentration. He works well in a small group, perhaps with just one other person. In a larger group he is liable to disturb others.

And, finally, with one staff member alone:

> He had a cuddle this morning. He tends to ask me how I am. He has his ups and downs.

Part of the diary procedure involved asking Jamie about his favourite people. The question was put in a way which allowed him to choose adults or children. He chose three other children, two boys and a girl. The reasons were similar in each case. They helped him out of trouble, and they were 'good friends'. In one case, Jamie helped his friend (with the goats).

When I had this picture of Jamie at Raddery, I went to see his mother at home. The discussion went back to a much earlier past when I asked about the reasons for Jamie's coming to Raddery and about his earlier schooling. I was told there had been problems ever since Jamie had started school. The difficulties, in her view, had been mainly at school but later they began to spill over into home. The mother said she had no relatives nearby to support her. Father worked away at sea in the oil industry.

At his last school, she said, Jamie had not only been abusive. He would 'swear and spit and attack people'. His head teacher had said he was 'a foul mouthed barbarian'. Raddery was seen by everyone concerned as 'a final solution, a last chance. No other school would take him'. She added 'We thought he was a lost cause'.

These seemed hard things to say but they were in the past. I asked mother about Jamie's future. She said until recently she had thought he might be unemployable. But she now knew he was possibly interested in catering courses. She wanted him to stay at Raddery until school leaving, as she could not see him settling in secondary school.

Finally, after I had seen the mother, and with her permission, I talked with the agency which had referred Jamie to Raddery, the local child guidance service. It seemed that originally Jamie had been referred to another child guidance service (in an area where the family had previously lived) by his mother because of his behaviour problems at home and settling in school after the summer holidays. But the later picture given by the mother of Jamie at school was confirmed. His behaviour had been described as 'intolerable' after an alternative primary school place had been carefully prepared for and tried.

Comprehensive psychological and neurological testing at this time showed that Jamie's intelligence was within the normal

range but that he had had some specific learning difficulties —
for example, a poor short-term memory. He had found it hard
to tolerate criticism at school.

The detailed picture of Jamie at school before he came to
Raddery was very different from the picture given by staff at
Raddery three to four years later. One can see only a pale
shadow of disagreeable behaviour where once it had all seemed
black. And the good side, the wish to be helpful to others, the
ability to be concerned even about a cause like Amnesty International, and the physical achievements in swimming as well
as the interest in cookery — all this had come about at Raddery.
This, in turn, had given a better picture of Jamie to his parents.
He looked forward to going home at weekends and his diary
shows he was helpful there too — stacking logs. And mother
could share a positive view of Jamie's future where once she had
thought him 'unemployable'.

In checking this material and obtaining permission to use it,
I was able to update the information nearly two years after the
diaries were kept.

Jamie has moved to Strathallan. Here staff hope he will
learn to take on more responsibility within the 'house' and within Raddery generally. These hopes are shared with his parents
whom I met at the Families Gathering in September 1990.

'Families Gathering' is an annual opportunity for parents
and others close to the child to meet other parents, as well as
staff, at Raddery. The children and staff prepare a kind of cele-
bration in the form of work children have done, which parents
can see at the school and there is usually a small entertainment.

I met Jamie's parents and little sister sitting at a table after
lunch in a marquee the school puts up for the occasion (in the
absence of a Hall which Raddery would like to build but for
which no funds are, as yet, available).

It was the first time I had met Jamie's father. After I introduced myself, his mother said: 'Jamie's come a long way' and
father immediately added:

> During the last couple of years he's come on. I can now
> get on with him. I used to feel I could knock his block
> off!

Mother reminded me that Jamie had been one of the children who had recently gone to the Soviet Union following the visit to Raddery of a group from the Leningrad special school (see Chapter 2). The parents had felt proud that he had been selected. 'I gave him everything he needed', father said.

I asked about the future. I was told Jamie would stay at Raddery until at least next Summer, doing work experience and English 'O' grade. 'He's got a target', mother said. They were pleased he had moved to Strathallan. It was good because it was a smaller unit. 'It will help him to become more of an individual' said father. He added his pleasure that Jamie had learnt to do his own washing and cooking. 'He is happier and more relaxed — though there are days when he's upset. But most people get upset sometimes'.

As one might expect in these circumstances, the parents had praise for what Raddery had contributed. 'We need more schools like this and teachers with the same understanding' said father, adding: 'He is considered as a normal child, not as a freak'. Mother added: 'If they had had more understanding (at previous schools) he might have been taught at an ordinary school. But they were out of their depth. They would rather ignore it and hope (the problem) would go away'. Father concluded by saying he couldn't say enough about Raddery and that Jamie had been so lucky to get a place there.

Meanwhile work with Jamie at Strathallan is continuing. He is attending a Youth Training Centre in a neighbouring town.

Jamie's story struck me as a practical illustration of the emphasis Raddery places on working to achieve harmony in children's lives in place of discord. Before he came to the school, there was only anger and resentment in his behaviour. There were similar feelings on the part of his parents because of their sense of failure. Now the processes were reversed. The parents were beginning to take pride in his achievements.

Paul

When I was first introduced to Paul, he was aged 14 and lived at Raddery's half-way house, Strathallan. He told me he had been at Raddery for over two years. He was previously at a secondary school and, before that, at a military services school — his father being in the Forces. He told me his father was coming out next year. At home he has a sister as well as his mother and father. His interests were aircraft and 'military stuff', reading, drawing and listening to records.

Paul was well able to keep his own diary without any assistance. He struck me as polite and somewhat reticent. His diaries were very full and he voluntarily kept them for a second week. They disclose not only events at Raddery and, at weekends, at home but also some of his feelings. Here are some of the entries:

> I went into my new class, but didn't go there (at first) because I thought there was a meeting. I settled down. After that I was with Alf. I was doing an experiment with sulphuric acid using zinc, a painted nail and an ordinary nail.

> At afternoon break I didn't bother going to have break. So I sat in the common room instead to wait for Paul [another child] to play me chess, because we agreed to play chess. Instead Adrian [staff] came and played me at chess. Paul was doing something else. After break I had Adrian for workshop.

> When my second class was finished I had to wait for the van [the school minibus that transports children between the school and Strathallan]. I didn't go to classes meeting. All of us at Strathallan had to have an early lunch because we were going to see a brass band. I enjoyed the brass band.

> [Later the same day] All at Strathallan had to have their tea quickly. We were going to help old folk. e.g. hold open the doors, with Jason [another child] and help push them in their wheelchairs. I enjoyed myself helping old folk.

[An expedition] The first plan was to drop one group of three. The first group me, Paul and Graham were dropped off at our spot. We then walked down to Lernie beach. You had to go through a forest footpath, then onto a path that brought you to a farm to get to the sea ... I really enjoyed it, throwing stones, collecting fossils (only Graham and Paul did). When we were picked up by Gerry and brought back all of us handed in our stuff. When it was over I wandered round. I met Kate [staff]. After a while I decided to go to class ... It was a good day.

After another expedition, hill-walking, Paul wrote:

After the expedition was finished, we went back to Raddery for senior meeting. It was a long, tiring but good hill walk. But I wish I could contribute to senior meeting.

I settled into some maths after break. I usually have difficulties with my maths but the difficulties may soon be over.

When lunch was over, went back to school. I had board games with Paul [staff]. It was fine at the start, but one boy got silly and that spoilt it for me.

Went for a drive in the van. Afterwards I was learning the guitar.

I had Spencer [staff] this morning for maths and that went well....

After the (afternoon) class finished Zoe and me had to go back down to Strathallan to cook the tea. When tea was complete and ready, Zoe and I had a game of table tennis. I enjoyed playing table tennis with Zoe.

This evening (various children named, 'except Zoe') went
to Avoch sports hall and played a game of badminton.

Other activities mentioned in the diaries include art 'doing a
self-portrait' and football.

The diaries also include a picture of week-ends spent at
home: 'When I came home I made my tea and watched tele-
vision. Later I played on the computer'. In answer to the diary
prompt 'Who were you with?' Paul wrote: 'Mum sometimes'.

There were events at home too:

Went out to a Christmas Party with Faith and Light — an
organization that looks after handicapped people — with
my mum, dad, sister and the rest of the Faith and Light
people. I didn't like the party much though the music
was good and I had difficulties joining in the dances and
staying awake.

During a different week-end at home, he played a family game,
which he enjoyed, and also made Sunday lunch with his sister.

When questioned further about his diary, Paul named only
one favourite or important person. This was his friend at
Raddery, Jason. They helped one another, he said. When I asked
him about his feelings for Jason, he said: 'A mixed bag. Sometimes we fall out and then we make it up. That's what is meant
by being best friends'.

His favourite activity at home was walking — 'better than
sitting around the house'. At Raddery he especially liked sports
and playing the guitar.

Unlike Jamie, there are no complaints from staff about
behaviour in Paul's case. During the time Paul kept diaries, staff
mainly commented on how helpful he was and considerate towards others. Comments also suggested progress he had made in
becoming more involved:

A super boy and an asset to the group because he doesn't
get involved in troublemaking. He now stands up for
other people in trouble. He was withdrawn and a bit
peculiar. He is now confident.

The other side of the problem of Paul's maths was given by Spencer. Spencer was worried and puzzled about his basic number concept. He was planning to involve him in peer tutoring with another boy.

In general, the comments suggested Paul underrated his own ability in other subjects. For example:

English three times a week. Most imaginative and creative boy in the school. Tremendous potential. Almost a zest for creative writing. Hard to square with his behaviour apparently at home. Interested in writing about flying. He has been able to learn concentration.

It was interesting that staff comments tended to be general about Paul and not related to any specific happenings during the week in question. It was as if he was only noticed over a period of time.

He is coming out of himself. He is beginning to make his own demands in his own quiet way. For example, he has actually asked to play something on his guitar. He will now instigate conversation. He has a sense of humour — quite subtle at times. His plan — well, we're beginning to see whether putting challenges in front of him will help him and he's beginning to meet them.

As with other children, the comments of staff he meets less often are interesting. For example:

I only see him if I'm doing break. If you're putting chairs around the tables, he always helps. He asks how you are. (Isobel, Domestic Bursar).

Asks how you are. Always chats to me. (Greta, House-worker).

Several staff referred to Paul's dramatic potential. Indeed, perhaps the staff only comment specific to the week being studied was that he 'gave a brilliant impression of an old tramp in the Friday meeting'.

The home visit I paid was with Paul's father and mother together. They were very ready to talk about their own family problems in relation to Paul's past difficulties. Mother had been very depressed when Paul was born on account of the death of another child. A third child died tragically later. In trying to get a picture of Paul from his parents before he came to Raddery, I saw him as someone very withdrawn who wouldn't speak to adults or to other children. He turned his back, even when talking to relatives. He had learning difficulties with regard to maths. His early schooling had been complicated by a move abroad because of his father's posting.

The parents had taken the initiative to refer Paul to the child guidance service as a means of getting him to Raddery. I correctly guessed, during the interview, that mother was a teacher. She saw Raddery as offering a secure environment which would help him to communicate, but, she said 'I was terrified at the thought'. Father said it had been a great relief to get him to Raddery. The parents described to me how their family relationships were complex and problematic and how this would have adversely affected Paul.

Progress in all sorts of ways was referred to. Paul could now travel by himself using public transport. He could manage money. They hoped he would stay on at Raddery and perhaps take advantage of training schemes. He had just had a very good interview with the Careers Advisory Service Officer. In general both parents were very pleased that Paul was opening out and developing,' in a way we had despaired of hoping would ever happen'.

As with Jamie, I followed this situation back to the referring agency (with permission). I was given a picture of Paul at primary school playground where he would live in a fantasy world of tanks, Star Wars, and so on, running around a corner of the playground on his own, imitating the sound of battle. Other children tended to ignore him. At secondary school, it seems, he avoided eye contact. It was difficult to have a straightforward conversation with him. He often responded with staccato phrases and inconsequential answers. Sometimes he seemed to have a mental block so that he could not answer at all. Yet Paul was described as surviving 'surprisingly well' at the Academy, spending most of his time in a small remedial class. But the psychologist felt there was a serious danger of his becoming psychotic without more intensive specialized help. She said that the kind of help available at Raddery was most likely to meet his needs.

In summing it up the psychologist said 'Life was exceptionally painful for Paul'. Yet he had come on at Raddery 'beyond anything that could have been imagined', although there were still some problems. The psychologist had been particularly impressed by Paul's performance in *Oliver* during the previous Families Gathering.

It is eighteen months later. Paul has left Strathallan and returned to live at home with his parents. I spoke to him on the telephone. His mother was out fetching his father from work. We had quite a long conversation. He told me he was attending a full-time Extension course at the local College of Further Education (FE) and he listed all the subjects he was doing. He was also attending the Air Training Corp (ATC) two evenings a week although he said that he had no intention of going into the services. Otherwise he could't think of much that he was doing. After reading to him the main parts of what I had written so far about him, I asked whether he had taking up drama or whether he was writing since leaving Raddery. No, he had not done any writing recently.

I asked Paul whether he missed Raddery. At first he said 'No', but a few moments later he added 'Sometimes I do have memories — I suppose I do miss it sometimes'. He told me about two friends he has — both Raddery youngsters who it is difficult to keep in touch with.

His parents came into the house while we were finishing our conversation, so I asked to speak briefly with mother. She told me that Paul had joined the ATC entirely on his own initiative and this was something he could never have done in the past. He had belonged to an ATC group when he was at Strathallan, but that was a much smaller group. She referred to this as part of the legacy of Raddery. Mother also told me that, in fact, Paul was doing pieces of writing to accompany comic strips — but he only showed them to a few people. He would do them if people asked for them.

Paul and Jamie are contrasting examples of children who have shown emotional development during their time at Raddery. Perhaps, what they have in common is their experience of healing and reconciliation with those closest to them as well as with society more generally.

It seems to me that in both cases progress has still to be consolidated. Paul is older and has accomplished a great deal in the light of earlier fears about his likely future. But now he has to manage without Raddery's intensive support. I shall be discussing the issues this raises in Chapter 8.

Angela

I move on next to the only girl in the sample who agreed to be included. She was an example of a child who only came to Raddery when she was 15 after failing to settle into ordinary secondary school.

Angela, was aged 16 when I met her and was already preparing to leave. On a typical morning she had work experience at a playgroup, and she enjoyed it. In the afternoon she was with 'The Oak House Group' and then at sport.

The 'Oak House' group is typical of the way spontaneity is blended with planned activities at Raddery. It happened that Christopher Fry (whose illustrations appear in this book) observed the interest Raddery children showed in his own children's Wendy House he had built in his front garden within the Raddery grounds. It is a place where Raddery children regularly passed by. Chris explained to me:

> The Oak House was my own idea which grew out of the Wendy house. The children saw it and this led to the idea. There are no constraints. It's a very solid structure but it's renewable. Children get security from it. It's deliberately using hardwood. I don't analyze it too much, but houses are important. They're where you live. It's the Three Little Pigs Syndrome.

Angela's diary recorded: '*I did enjoy it*'.

Another feature of Angela's diary is that it shows the mutual support between herself and other older children. On one occasion, she invited another girl to her house. On another evening she went on a birthday walk with a group of children and got covered with eggs, toothpaste and water. 'Yes, I enjoyed myself'. Again, another evening was spent 'playing football and darts with all my friends', which was 'quite good fun'.

At the week-end on a Saturday Angela was 'away with my mother up town to spend my birthday money'. In the afternoon she was with a Raddery friend in town. In the evening she went on a trip to Cromarty with a group from the school.

On Sunday: 'I was in the bedroom most of the morning. I was with — (my friend). It was boring'. In contrast 'This afternoon I was playing football matches. There were crowds of people. It was brilliant!' In the evening she was in Sunday meeting: 'It was kind of boring, except when Gerry's music started to play'.

So the diary tells us that Angela is a sociable person who has found varied ways to enjoy life with others. In contrast, her diary explains that she dislikes attending Raddery's many meetings.

The staff comments for the corresponding week in general paint a picture of a girl, who had her 17th birthday during the week, somewhat fatigued with Raddery and with school during her final year:

> She feels she has done it. There was an incident on Friday when, as a change from routine work, I asked her to type letters and see this through by putting them onto the word processor. Secondly, I asked her to make a list of shops which might take adverts for the (Raddery) magazine. She refused, saying: 'I'm not your slave — give me some English work to do'. She shouted. Eventually she did do some English as an alternative.

Again, from a different staff member:

> She was upset on one occasion last week. She was swearing. I talked in a motherly way and put my arm around her and talked to her very quietly. She had been arguing with another girl and another member of staff was calming her. I can't remember what it was about.

But other staff confirm her sociability and also her physical prowess:

> I see her for football. She is excellent. She is strong and skilful — on a par with the best boys. She had played before she came to Raddery.

Some of the problems staff face with Margaret seem to be within the range of fairly normal behaviour for someone of that age:

> She goes down weekly to Rosemarkie for work experience. She is said to be super with the kids. There is a tempest inside her. She gets jealous with other children. She erupted last Thursday night. She was making a noise in the common room and staff talked to her. She couldn't accept it. She said she wouldn't go to bed and I said she had to. In the end I had to sit on her to prevent her from hurting herself. After a time I got up and said: 'you're an adult. You can do what you want to calm down.' She went for a walk with Alison [child] and came back after a while okay. There are never any repercussions after an incident like this. She likes to be the boss — the top dog. For two years she has been the fire officer. I recently asked her to go round the whole of Raddery checking up the equipment and she did this very responsibly. She can organize a fire practice herself.

A visit to Angela's home — where I met Angela on the step shortly after she had left Raddery — enabled me also to talk with her mother. The household comprised herself, Angela and Angela's younger sister. It was the kind of area where there was lots of coming and going with neighbours — even while I was there. Mother told me that Angela had been attending a local children's centre before she went to Raddery. From the schooling point of view, mother said there had only been problems at the secondary stage, where Angela had been expelled.

When I came to update the picture of Angela some eighteen months later, I was told she had left Raddery, returned home and later given birth to a baby. I called at her mother's house. Her sister met me at the door and told me where I would find her. She had left her parents and moved in with a lady in the next street. She was not at home there either but I was told she was visiting in the house on the corner with 'fish tanks in the window'. This turned out to be her uncle's house. Angela met me and warmly welcomed me in. She showed me her baby, fast asleep in beautifully clean clothes in a nice pram. She was beaming as I praised her baby — a boy. Things were going fine. She thought it was better for her to live away from her mother. It was a very brief visit as I was catching a train but I said I would call again and she said I would be very welcome.

Again, the story of Angela raises questions about what happens after children leave which I shall discuss in Chapter 8.

The next two children to be introduced are examples of younger children who continued to present problems as well as to make progress during the two years I was collecting material for this book.

David

David was 12 years old when I first met him and had already been at Raddery for two years. He told me his interests were swimming, football and TV. Asked about the most important people in his life, he first of all quickly said his mum, dad and sister but then gave a second answer comprising two staff (male) and one child (female) at Raddery. He could only manage his diary for one day.

His 'team-mate', Paul (staff) explained what may have been the problem:

On Monday there was a difficulty. He was told to have his meal out of the dining room by Bill. He went to his bedroom and tipped the food out. I put him in the porch where he stayed and where we could keep an eye on him. He had done something like throw a chair that morning. During the preceding week he had tried not to go home. I told him it was too late. Earlier he had been okay about going home and looked forward to it. The family seemed to be unsettled.

Other staff members also told me about his not wanting to go home. He usually goes home two week-ends out of three but suddenly he had not wanted to go this week-end.

Some staff thought that David had generally improved recently. For example:

He's improved during the last few weeks. He has a problem in that he is rude to kitchen staff. He had hoped to be in the kitchen group for jobs but David Dean had taken him off because of bad behaviour and he's had to think about this. It has helped to focus attention on him and that is maybe why he has improved.

Another staff member commented:

We keep re-inforcing his strengths. His language is shocking. Last Thursday night I told their dormitory (the largest with five children) a story to calm them down. The aim is to help him to be reasonable with people.

Like Angela, David is a keen football player. One member of staff at Strathallan said this helps to maintain what she calls a 'lightness to the relationship' since they support different teams. 'Other relationships David has with adults are pretty serious and to do with his problems'.

At home, David has his mother and father, an older sister and a baby sister. I only met his mother who spoke of previous schooling as a disaster. She said the school tried. He had a one-to-one teaching situation with a special teacher, 'But it didn't work. He used to roll under the table swearing'.

Mother explained how she and her husband did not want David to go to Raddery at first. At the time, after a social worker had been brought in and they had visited the school, they said they had 'reluctantly accepted it'. Now she recognized there had been progress. She said he used to be more highly strung. She said she was quite happy with the way he was coming on.

David continued to improve for a while. At one point they had been considering introducing him into mainstream school. But this had made him feel threatened and his behaviour and problems then became worse.

The Raddery staff had more recently tried to understand David's difficulties at a deeper level. Visits were paid to the home in co-operation with the Social Work Department. The parents were helpful in sharing information about their own problems when David had been a baby. They had separated several times and the mother had been extrememly depressed.

In the light of what was learnt, it was decided that David should be one of the children selected for the new *Cottage* venue opened in September 1990. Here he is getting closer attention in a smaller group, protected during large parts of the day from the difficulties of being with larger numbers of other people. Graeme Mochrie, the team leader at the *Cottage*, told me attempts had been made to build up the relationship — from both sides — between David and his mother. But the summer holidays had not been too good and although he had generally settled in the *Cottage* after the holidays there had been an serious incident with a lady member of staff.

I spoke to David briefly in a corner of the marquee during the Families Gathering 1990. His parents had not been able to attend (although they lived fairly locally). This could not have been too easy for him on an occasion when almost all the other children had their folks with them. I also knew that in the preceding weeks he had had mixed feelings about talking again to me about the book. So I was glad to be able to read to him what I had written and allow him to comment. I agreed to leave out mention of one past problem he wanted left out but otherwise, he said, it was okay but he couldn't stay and talk to me any longer.

Warren

Warren was 12 years old when I first met him. At that time he had been at Raddery just over a year. He told me he lived at home with his mother and father, younger sister and younger brother. His favourite activities were art, the Oak House and 'morning classes'. He named two favourite people, both of them other Raddery children. His reasons for chosing them were that they helped him. Of one he said 'He calms me down and tells me not to get into trouble'. Of his other choice he said 'He helps with problems'. In both instances, Warren said he helped his friends similarly. Warren's diary was well kept although the entries were very brief. The morning activities he apparently liked included reading, geography and maths. Reading featured particularly prominently: 'I did maths and then I did reading'. 'Read a library book'.

Afternoon activities included the Oak House, art, football, craft (which he also told me he liked), swimming, and drama. There were very few comments but for one evening when he went for a walk he wrote 'I was being abusive'. On another evening he did science and he commented 'I enjoyed making a candle'. He also commented that he enjoyed art and maths. Cooking was mentioned, but there was no comment.

The following were some comments from staff:

He does good quality creative writing. He has good basic competence for his age. He was happy in his work this week and more ready to relate to me.

I used to clean his room but he has moved to a different room. He has been awfully nice this week. He can be hostile. I try to be the same all the time. I asked about the times when he was not so nice. I was told he tends to say 'Shut up: get out of the way'. But, I was told, 'The cross bits don't last long'.

I have him for craft work. He was more quiet than normal. Sometimes he has a language problem, i.e. foul language. I had a meal with him. He was exceedingly pleasant and relaxed.

He treats me with ambivalence. He has real difficulties at home. I represent home. He gave me some small toys he wanted me to keep safe. I accepted this. I thought this was about secret knowledge — his parents had been going to split up and now finally had split up. There is a Social Worker in touch.

In my class for primary language work, reading and writing and maths. He is interested but a bit unsettled in class. Nothing serious happened last week but he lacks concentration. For example, there are flying rubbers, silly noises, swinging on chairs and fiddling with elastic bands. This has been noted at a previous team meeting for attention. But he has been better than he used to be and therefore there were no strong measures for his misdemeanours.

I have to check his behaviour but then I also can talk with him about candle-making and electronics. We will come up here and make candles. This is voluntary. He made candles last week.

He is very keen on drama. He is a good cameraman.

I am his team mate. I am also his acting team leader. I contacted his mother over the week-end. Father had just left home. I was concerned that he might be seen by mother to be taking father's place with his macho attitudes. I have been able to talk to Warren about his feelings and while he had said about his father 'I feel angry but I don't hate him'. I feel mother still needs help and I will phone her again.

Because I knew there had been a family crisis I left it for several months before visiting. I then saw his mother. Compared with other children, they live relatively close to Raddery. The mother told me she had been married three times. The brother and sister Warren had told me about are in fact half-brother and half-sister. Mother said she was in the process of getting her third divorce. Warren's step-father, whom he calls 'Dad', comes to visit the house on Sundays and likes to take Warren out shopping. Warren likes to be taken out but sometimes tears his clothes on the way home to make sure that father buys new ones. It struck me that the family were probably poor and that father would have to buy all the new clothes. I asked mother whether problems at school or at home had lead to Warren going to Raddery and she said 'Both'. At school he wouldn't do lessons and he caused damage either to children or to furniture. At home he was the same. He used to damage furniture and carpets. He had moods within himself rather than moods which were reactive. Mother told me she had been to see a psychiatrist when he was 7 years old. The psychiatrist said he would be okay — and he was okay for a week! She spoke highly of the social worker who had moved to a local children's centre and had let it be known that she could turn to her any time she wanted.

Mother told me that holidays are a problem. Warren will be home for two weeks and then spend one week at the children's centre followed by two weeks at home in order to break the summer holiday up. Although there may be improvements insofar as Warren is concerned at school — at least during the week when he kept a diary — problems at home continue. Mother told me of one recent incident. He had thrown salt into his sister's eyes. He said it was an accident but mother told him it clearly wasn't an accident and he flew into a temper. She said he takes about an hour to come out of his moods and then he sidles up to her and to apologize ... She can tell when his mood is over. About the future, mother said she hoped he would stay at Raddery until he was 16. She said his ambition used to be 'going on the dole', but more recently this had changed and he wanted to be in the Royal Air Force (RAF). She doubted if the RAF would have him. It was clear, meantime, that Warren was happier at Raddery then at home. I asked about his relationships with his brother and sister. Mother said he used to hate his sister but recently he will now talk to her and play with her. He just sees his brother as a nuisance. When I asked about any other friends I was told he does have two friends in his old school but he doesn't now see much of them. He tends to stay at home. Some of the neighbours are a bit standoffish and won't speak to him. Mother thought Warren now had more insight into his difficulties and she said this is what the school has done for him.

About eighteen months after this interview, I met mother at Families' Gathering 1990. By this time, with the introduction of separate 'venues' (see page 25, Chapter 2) Warren had moved to the *Cottage*. A group of us met round the small dining-room table there — mother, grand-parents, sister, brother, a member of staff and Warren himself. It was a social occasion where everybody seemed to be avoiding saying what they really felt, so I arranged to extricate firstly Warren and then his mother to talk to them individually in another room.

I knew from Graeme Mochrie, Warren's new team leader at the *Cottage*, that things had not gone too well over the summer, although at school he was 'mainly trying hard'. Graeme referred to an 'underlying unhappiness' which sometimes expressed itself in destructiveness or defiance, although at other times 'he can relax'.

He was fairly relaxed when I spoke with him, despite our having to stand while we talked in a small spare room where there was nowhere to sit down — other rooms being filled with visitors at the Gathering.

When I asked how things were, he said quietly 'Much the same'. He said he preferred to be at the *Cottage*. He welcomed the fact that, as he put it, 'They keep an eye on you. They pick you up on everything'. With a 1:1 staff:child ratio at the *Cottage*, this is very true and I knew from what Graeme had told me that Warren knew very well why he had been selected for the *Cottage* when children had been allocated to the different 'venues' in the summer.

Warren then told me he expected to be at the *Cottage* for a year. This was because Mr Dean had told him 'there would be different children in a year's time'. (This was true. It was precisely what David Dean had said to encourage the *Cottage* children to believe that he expected movement. Warren had taken it to heart).

I asked Warren what his hopes were for the future. He reminded me he was 14 years old. He said he would stay at Raddery until he was 16 years old and then he wanted to be a technician. A problem, he said, was holidays. They went 'on and on and on and on'.

When I interviewed mother (in the same surroundings) a few minutes later she agreed with this last statement, although she didn't express it quite like Warren had! A local children's centre is still used for holiday respite. 'He doesn't tell me a lot', she said — although she knew he enjoyed being in the *Cottage*. She recognized there had been some progress: 'He is more responsible in himself. He stops and thinks before he does things and he understands himself a lot better than he ever did'. Mother also felt it was better for Warren at home because his father no longer called. 'But', she said, 'we still face a lot of problems'.

It seemed to me that mother was happier in herself than when I had first met her after the crisis of her divorce. But what now impressed me was that both mother and Warren were beginning to develop an understanding of each other.

Mother praised what Raddery was doing. 'I'm glad the school's here', she said. 'I really am glad'. But she said she had one 'comment', as she called it. She said there were so many activities at Raddery that couldn't be done at home — and certainly not in their home. The implication was that it was very hard to keep a lively boy occupied at home in the kinds of ways he was accustomed to at Raddery.

Finally, I asked mother if she thought what was being done for Warren at Raddery could have been accomplished at an ordinary school. She replied:

> No. He was chucked out of two of them. And I could not have got through to him in the way that Raddery staff can.

In her concise matter-of-fact way, I felt she had told me a great deal. I will be taking up in later chapters the point about following the Raddery levels of activity in more modest home surroundings as well as her answer to my question about an ordinary school.

David and Warren both illustrate the closeness of home experiences to children even while they are living at Raddery.

I will next trace the history of two children who had moved from the main school to Strathallan. In the autumn of 1990, when my period of gathering material was coming to a close, one of them, Jonathan had recently left and returned home. The second child, John, was still at school but his future, relating closely to the situation at home, was uncertain.

Jonathan

Jonathan was aged 15 when I first saw him towards the end of 1988. He had already come to Strathallan from the main school. He had a serious problem with his eyesight and diary keeping was not easy, but he managed with support from staff. His favourite activities, he told me, were computing, TV (both at home and at school) and playing an electric keyboard — which he can also do at home and at school. His important friends were a member of Raddery staff and two mates at home. He did not name any children at Raddery. He lives in a small town a long way from Raddery. His diary tells of his school programme and also of his daily living at Strathallan:

Got up, had breakfast. Did bread and papers.

Stayed in watched the telly. Laid my table. Went to bed.

Morning meeting. Two classes. Dinner. Gerry for music. Kate for music. Home for tea.

Watched the box. Played dominoes. Out for walk. Drink then diary.

Went for walk. Watched the box. Had telephone call from Mum and Dad. Then bed.

With the exception of music and art, he gave the names of his teachers rather than the subjects:

> First class Spencer. Second class Alf.

The diary continued into the week-end, spent at home, where a few more details were included than for days at Raddery:

> Got pack lunch. Went back to school (from Strathallan) Went to community meeting then free time then caught a train from ... to ... then to ... (home town). Played badminton with Dad. Got home. Played pool. Listened to music. My dad stepped back and hurt his calf muscle playing badminton.

> Got up 11.0 am. Watch the box and had breakfast.

> Went out to (friend's) house and watched videos. Had tea then out again.

> (Sunday) Out all afternoon working (with friend).

> Went to (local hotel) to see High Spirits (with Mum, Dad and friend). Back home played pool with Mum and watched *Cell Block D*.

Staff comments for the same week help us to develop a portrait of Jonathan:

> Difficult to get close to. Distant. Not the type one can get close to. Not working in class and therefore having to do overtime. He had to stay in the preceding Saturday for this. He went home last week-end. This was okay. He doesn't show his emotions.

I wondered if the last remark was generally true or whether he was very careful and cautious before he made friends. He told me, for example, that his friends at home with whom he was close were lads he had known for many years.

He gets one-to-one help from Morag (part-time staff). He has an eye defect. He is under-achieving and therefore we are trying to edge him forward on all fronts to give him stimulus in class to increase his motivation. His eye condition will worsen. He is best in discussion work, oddly enough (because of his eyesight difficulty) after watching TV.

Another staff member referred to his move to Strathallan:

Has had a honeymoon period (at Strathallan) until recently. This is now over. He tends to sit in front of TV all night.

Several members of staff referred to his lack of enthusiasm for activities. For example:

There was a tiff with him recently at the Oak House. He turned up and when I said he was coming to work here he said 'Yes, worst luck!' I asked him what he would like to do and he replied 'As little as possible'. I made him go away for two minutes and then, when he came back, he worked okay.

When I visited Jonathan's family home I discovered that both parents worked and that Jonathan is an only child. The discussion was friendly, with father periodically disagreeing with what mother said. Mother said she was first aware that something was 'wrong' when Jonathan was at playschool. He was hyperactive, mother said — though father didn't agree with that term. On one occasion mother had mistakenly left a bottle of tranquillisers out where Jonathan could reach them. He helped himself to a large dose after spilling them out on the floor. As a result, he was more hyperactive than ever, she thought! He also used to wander off as a toddler. They had contacted 'the welfare officer' who had told them to 'let him wander'. Mother said they had thought this was strange advice, but that they had better do what the welfare officer said. They were worried when he wandered out of sight but, mother said, he always landed up with other children.

At primary school he would 'niggle' other children. He lacked bowel control (a problem which was to recur later). He was referred to the psychiatric ward of a children's hospital. Father said his schoolwork improved there but mother said the experience was a failure. At all events, he was transferred to another psychiatric hospital. In discussing the various schools he had tried, mother said: 'If he could have had a school without children he'd have done fine!'

The parents told me he was referred to Raddery because he could not cope with secondary school. He had liked the idea because he had been told it was 'voluntary'. (This is true in the sense that children are not normally sent to Raddery under compulsory orders). Jonathan had taken this to mean he didn't have to go!

When we got on to the Raddery staff who had said Jonathan was lazy, it was clear mother wanted to identify with him. It was not that he minded doing things so much as that sometimes he thought it was just that he should be asked. Father interjected to say I had been asking what they, as parents thought, not what Jonathan felt. Then mother told me there had been benefits. He had offered to help when mother had been hard-pressed preparing a meal. Father said he had also 'nearly volunteered' to clean the windows — though here mother contradicted father to say he hadn't volunteered because father had asked him. Father then explained the point he was trying to make was that he had not ordered him to do it. At all events, it was clear he had been more willingly helpful recently in the house.

We talked about Jonathan's future. He could stay an extra year at Raddery. The problem with his eyesight is that he has optical atrophy. Most of the things he is keen on, he cannot do. So work will be a problem. The parents assumed he would be coming back to live with them at home when he leaves Raddery.

Two years' later I renewed contact. Jonathan had left Strathallan and Raddery to return home. Jonathan had now been registered as partially sighted. When I asked him about this he said it was 'the only thing I could do really'. Father, to whom I spoke afterwards on the phone, put it more positively. An employer would have to know anyway about his poor eyesight, he said, and it was better to be 'up front with it'. I learnt that Jonathan had been on an eight-week assessment course (in the nearest city) and that he now had YTS employment with an electrical company. He was hoping to go to college soon to take a course in computing.

Jonathan sounded cheerful. I asked him about his friends and I suggested that perhaps he was quite unusual in keeping close friends at home during the four years he had been at Raddery. He replied: 'Yes, and a few new friends'. Further questions and answers led to his saying that he had a girlfriend and 'a few mates'. He also told me of various hobbies — cycling occasionally, keyboard instruments, computing — as well as watching TV and videos.

I then asked him if he missed Raddery (which he had left four months previously). Without hesitation he replied:

Not Raddery, but I miss Strathallan. I miss the friends
I had there.

He told me he would be paying a visit to see his friends again. But, he said, he had been able to keep in touch with them on the telephone.

I then asked Jonathan's father to comment on the contribution that Raddery had made to Jonathan's progress — progress which father readily acknowledged. He had mixed views. While he recognized the contrast between Jonathan as he was now and Jonathan as he had once been, he thought it was 'a pity he had to be away from home so much — although that did relieve the pressure a bit at home'.

I followed up this telephone call with a final visit. Jonathan sat next to his father on a settee and mother close by while the draft pages from this book were passed from father to mother and then back to Jonathan. We went over a few details and clarified a few points. It all seemed so harmonious that I said I wondered if I had exaggerated about the extent to which mother and father had disagreed in the past. Father assured me I had been absolutely accurate — and mother accepted that! While father and mother read every word carefully, Jonathan — whose poor eyesight meant it was harder for him to keep up with the reading — said he would read it when the book came out.

John

John was aged 14 when I first met him at Raddery. He explained to me that he lived mostly with his step-mother and father, but that he also spent some time with his mother and step-father. He said he had a half brother living with father and a sister living with mother. He had been at Raddery for one and a half years. He had previously been in ordinary schools and attending a special teaching centre. He had some difficulty in answering when I asked about his interests. He mentioned computing. He did not keep a diary for me but we had quite a clear picture of him at Raddery from staff. For example, Christopher Fry told me:

> Three times a week he is working at the Oak House. He has a remarkable way of thinking which is very interesting. I am not myself a carpenter. John can see things creative which I can't see. It's as though it were lateral thinking. For example, if you give up on a particular tool to do a particular job John will find a way round. In the evenings I played chess with him. He is very good and completely unpredictable. He doesn't see very many moves ahead, but enough.

> He is a 'touchy' boy. He has disgusting table manners. I can be authoritative with him even though there was a different kind of relationship when we are building the Oak House. We do everything at the Oak House from drawing the plans to painting. I also see John out of hours — for example, last week. They play at the Oak House then too. It's a bit of an excuse for letting kids play in a meaningful way — they create their own fantasies.

Another member of staff told me of an incident where John had objected to David Dean's new policy of checks on classrooms. He got caught and it wasn't fair! He has his own moral code. He walked out. He was prevented from actually leaving by David and Bill. John was also described as self-centred and inward-looking.

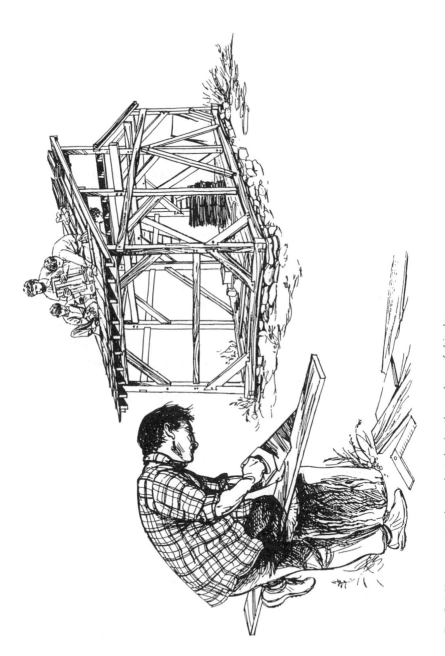

The Oak House construction project: Laying the cedar roof shingles.

One of the teachers who does number work with John said:

> He wants to be over-helpful. He manages to stop himself
> sometimes, e.g. 'I don't know if you wanted me to do
> that'. He has a need to try to do things for adults. He is
> intelligent and able to do things in the right way.

Another of the teachers told me:

> I have him in class for Standard Grade Science. He needs
> encouragement to apply himself. Science is something he
> is keen on and wanting to know about at times. At other
> times I have to push him.

John is also described as a 'competent swimmer' who 'listens to
instructions'. 'At the end of formal sessions we have great fun
which he loves for about 10–15 minutes'.

Another comment was that 'he knows what work is about.'

> He has recently moved to his present class. He has one
> full year and a bit to go for Standard Grade exams. He
> is a slow but competent reader. His writing skills are
> weaker. He has recently been writing a longish story
> some of it published in the *Raddery Rag*.

So John comes across as likeable to staff in many ways and as
someone who needs a range of relationships with different staff.
He also has more academic potential than many Raddery children may have.

With this picture in my mind, I visited John's father and
step-mother. As with some of the other children, he lives a long
distance away from Raddery in a small town. The father told me
John had attended the local primary school before the family
split up. He then went to the local school where his mother
lived. There were apparently some incidents which led to his
coming before the Children's Hearing. As a result he was returned to his father and to his old primary school. Again there
were difficulties. Father said it was 'like running into a brick
wall'. It was then that he attended a local special learning class.

The father said he had hoped John would go to the local secondary school and they had an interview with the head teacher. However, the school would not take him. The father saw this as being because his academic standards were not high enough. They were then given the choice of two special schools and they chose Raddery because they thought the alternative would allow him to mix with other children who might get him into trouble with 'glue sniffing and minor drugs'. Also the alternative school, father thought, was too near and he could be 'up and off and skip school and come home'.

The father, who is an engineer, had no enormous expectations of Raddery. He told me he had been amazed when he had been shown round the school by a girl pupil who had been so full of praise for the school. He said he thought this was unusual for a child to be keen on her own school. When I asked father what he expected of Raddery for the future for John, he replied carefully: 'To make him more responsible for himself, pointing him in the right direction, how to go about finding a job, interviewing, filling in forms and facing up to his own responsibilities'.

A year and a half later, I made contact with John again. He had moved from the main school to Strathallan. John told me that in some ways he missed living at the main school because there was less to do in the evenings at Strathallan. But he enjoyed his work experience with a local bakery. He would like to work in a bakery and he told me his mother had said there was currently a vacancy in a bakery in his home town.

This last interview with John occurred at a time of crisis. It was the day before the half-term break and John told me he was not sure where he was going to stay or whether he was going to come back. I learnt later that the uncertainty was in part provoked by the school in trying to help John to face up to some decision-making about his future. John talked freely with me about his past. For example, he filled in the details about how he had come before the Children's Hearing. He had raided an ice-cream van and made off with the takings. He said he was glad he had come to Raddery because when he met up during home visits with past friends who had gone to the ordinary secondary school 'I see all the trouble I would have got into'.

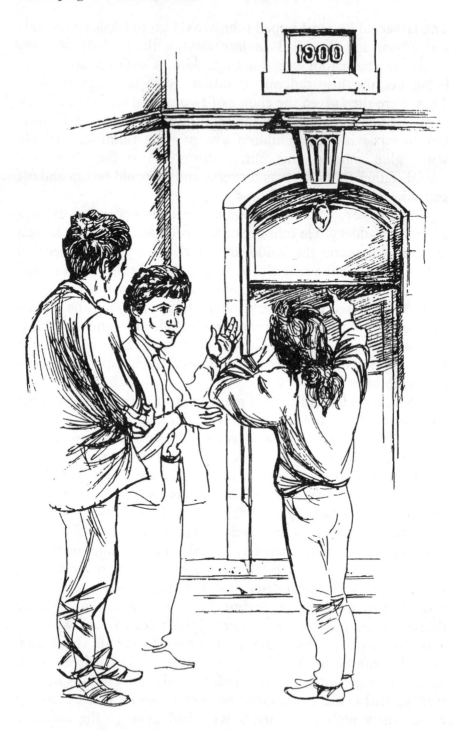

A child shows visiting parents around the school.

John said would prefer to stay at Raddery until the end of the school year — in about nine months' time. I suggested that, for purposes of his future plans, we assume he was staying. In this case, I asked, what view of the future did he have? He repeated that he would like to work in a bakery and there was a possibility he could attend a bakery course at the College Further Education in Inverness.

We also talked about the talent he had for what Chris Fry had called 'lateral thinking'. He acknowledged with a smile that he knew what I meant. I asked if he missed Chris (who had left Raddery). He said 'Not as much as I miss Gerry' (another staff member who had left more recently). He told me he had tried recently to contact Gerry.

I later learnt that staff at Strathallan were concerned that John needed to be pushed to take responsibility for preparing to leave and that a lot of work was being put into this. There would be problems for him if he returned either to mother or to father. The likely outcome of the present crisis would be that he would stay at Strathallan until the end of the school year and that the staff would work intensively with him to prepare for the future.

George

Finally I will describe George, a child who left Raddery fairly soon after I had first made contact with him in 1988.

George told me he was aged 15 and had been at Raddery for two years. He had come from another special school which was nearer to his home in a Scottish city. He told me that at home were his father, step-mother and sister. At Raddery, he said, his interests included skiing, swimming and football and he also liked swimming and football at home. At home, too, he told me, he had a dog.

George had difficulty with his writing, but he thought he could ask a staff-member (his team-mate) to keep his diary for him. In the event, this did not happen, so we have no diary! However, I did talk with him again in more detail about the activities and people he liked best. To football he added, this time, 'workshop' and 'work experience'. I later learnt from staff that he was doing metal work. I was told he would try even though he made constant mistakes. He was better at work experience than at the workshop at Raddery because there was less distraction from other children. In answer to my question, whether this could lead to employment, his instructor said he could find a job as a gas welder but 'he would have to learn to concentrate more'.

From a different perspective, Betty, the Raddery House-keeper, reported that she had told George that she admired a flower stand he had made in the metal workshop. He was 'absolutely delighted' and she ended up buying it!

So far we have seen George in a positive light — 'a likeable boy', as Yvonne, the assistant cook, put it. But a boy does not transfer from one special school to another, many miles away, for nothing! So, let the picture unfold from some other staff comments:

> Flares up but now comes out of it very quickly. Had a fight with William [child] on Wednesday. He has a violent and rapid reaction, typical of many Raddery children. He needs holding and calming and gently brow-beating out of it.

> His last year at school. He is very practical. He has a very short concentration span. He is easily distracted and influenced by other children who, themselves, have learning difficulties. His reading is very basic.

> He is having a difficult spell. There was one incident when another staff member had made him stand in a room where I was. My part was simply to support the other staff member. I told him he had to stay there until the other staff member came to tell him he could go. He was standing in the corner swearing. Eventually the other staff person came in and told him to keep a civil tongue or he would stay there longer.

Comes in Monday, Wednesday and Friday for number work. There was a fracas on Friday but he was peripheral to this.

He used to steal and then, when getting out of this, used to pretend to steal.

He attends for a food and nutrition class. This is a small class [four]. He is usually in high spirits. He gets on with things. However, he thinks cooking is 'woman's work'.

I'm his team leader. I try to keep him out of his sullen moods. This is when he gets into trouble with other kids, e.g. name calling. We try to keep a general eye on him and steer him out of possible complaints.

I am his team mate. No class contact. I see him on a day-to-day basis. For example: Thursday night. He can go down to the level of little kids. We try to drag him out of this to act the age he is. He biffed a younger child who needled him. He doesn't settle to things. We have to try to keep him out of trouble. He smokes. He uses bizarre language. He doesn't have a close friend, yet he is usually well liked. He has had three foster-parents and many schools — Raddery is the only one that has not failed.

George himself did not say he was without close friends. He described his friendships towards three Raddery children, top of the list being Sofia. 'You can depend on her', he said. 'When she was in trouble, she let you help her'. Another child, a boy, was described as 'a natural friend'.

It was some months later before I managed to visit George's father and, by this time, George had left Raddery. He was immersed with his street mates, and had to be called in by his father to say 'hello'. I hardly recognized the George I knew from Raddery. I wondered if here smoking, at least, if not foul language and violent behaviour could be the norm in the neighbourhood? Yet clearly there had been other more personal problems.

The father readily enlightened me. He introduced me to his second wife with whom, he said, he had now been living for eight years. He explained that his first marriage had been a disaster. There was drunkenness and violence and fighting. His first wife had become a prostitute. This marriage broke up when George was aged 6. Father moved to another city. George and his sister went into ₁ children's home and were then fostered. However, George's foster placement broke down and, according to father, the foster parents 'bruised him'. It was easier for his sister. George was 'a rough and tumble boy'. Eventually he returned home and attended ordinary school. But he was disturbing other children and was sent to the local special school. 'Things didn't work out. He was pinching bicycles and taking them to his mother who, at that time, was living at a caravan site'.

Father compared the local special school with Raddery in terms of George's attitudes to it. He would not get up in the morning to return to the local school (where he was also a boarder). But he would get up early when it was time to go to Raddery and say 'I'm off'. He didn't settle at first at Raddery, however. There were tears in his eyes when he went the first time because he thought he was going into care. When he came back, he said 'It's great'. There was an improvement after two to three terms.

I asked about work for George. The father explained that Raddery had been prepared for George to stay a further year. But George wanted to leave (to be more 'grown-up'?). Father said he let George decide. He'd hoped he could have a course in welding — or perhaps Raddery had hoped this — where he lived, but nothing had materialized. So he does odd jobs with his father.

It is not easy from the stories of Jamie and Paul, Angela, or Warren and David, or from the accounts of Jonathan and John or George — to reach any single conclusion about what the

Raddery experience has meant for them. They have varied backgrounds, individual personalities and they are at different stages of development. The optimistic point is that with each of them there has been movement since they first came to Raddery. In some instances this contrasts with a sense that they were stuck before they came to Raddery.

In a deeper sense, I think it is too soon to evaluate their experiences. Surely, it is only years afterwards that most of us can really evaluate our school years — especially if, as in my own case, some of this time was spent in residential settings? In my case, I spent a year, aged 10, in a residential boarding school on account of the war and, after returning to day school until the age of 12, the rest of my schooling, through my own choice and my father's income, was spent in residential schools. I am still, more than forty years on, trying to work out for myself some aspects of what this meant.

Certainly for me, as for each of the children at Raddery, there was much unfinished educational and emotional business still to be attended to when I left.

One point I find myself almost taking for granted, because I know Raddery so well, is the value the children generally place on being at the school — and perhaps especially when they reach the stage of being at Strathallan. This does not mean that they love every moment of it. They are quite often unhappy or worried and sometimes, like all children, bored. Their understanding of why they are at Raddery, however, and of how other children as well as adult staff can help them is in many instances remarkable.

The same is true of the parents.

Parents' Views about Raddery

Parents tended to have a clear understanding of Raddery's role, often expressed succinctly. In particular they recognized the need to combine dealing with problems and offering education. As one parent put it, Raddery aimed 'to sort his behaviour and then to give him the schooling'.

Another parent saw Raddery in terms of offering a friendly, more free environment than the normal school. Some parents expressed concern about the education side of the school. They were anxious that their children were not losing out educationally by being at Raddery. One parent complained that she didn't know enough about her child's progress educationally.

Other parents emphasized security. Raddery offered a secure environment which would 'help him to communicate with other kids. It would be less threatening for him and he would get some peace'.

All the parents expressed praise for the staff. For example:

> The teachers knew what they were fighting against with the kids. She compared this with (a children's home) where, she claimed the teachers were not qualified enough.

Another parent told me:

> The way they work has to be seen to be believed. I have seen them doing it. They have patience.

And again:

> They are totally integrated as a staff team. They plan things. They are in it altogether. They are all in the plan. It is integration at its best.

I asked parents about a number of specific aspects of the school. These were standard questions I had used in research into special education at a number of other schools. One of these questions was about the understanding the school had for the problems faced by parents — an issue where the other schools I had studied did not always score very highly.*

---

* See, for example, SEED, P: *Children with Profound Handicaps — Parents Views and Integration.* Falmer Press, 1988.

They are always ready to listen.

Very understanding. When she started going to Raddery, my problems stopped with her.

One parent who had a criticism in answer to my question linked this with the distance the school was from home. She said 'There is a distance barrier'.

Reviews was another topic which, in other research, has raised controversy with parents. The general view of parents at Raddery was favourable but there were a variety of comments. For example:

I am not sure about the benefit of reviews. I attend about every six months. It depends on what you mean by helpful. They come out with certain suggestions they think might help. I just sit and listen to what he has been doing. They suggested he should have more help from the educational psychologist but I don't know if anything came of this.

Again:

There was a difference between the first and second review. On the first occasion they (parents) had detailed written reports. On the second occasion they were concentrating on what he was going to do when he left school.

And:

It's useful to get ... [child] sitting there. He is brought into it but most of the things I find out I know already.... the great thing is that ... [child] is involved. They give us something else to work on.

But another parent said:

I have a low opinion of the last review. It was a waste of time. It was a waste of money. They only told me what I already knew. We are due for a review this coming week and the social worker is taking us there.

One topic on which parents commented very favourably was the range of activities available at Raddery including major events like summer camps. For example:

> He looks forward to activities like summer camps. There is nothing like that that could continue now he has left school. He was not a sporty type before he went to Raddery but his interests have broadened. He doesn't tell us what's happening until afterwards. For example, we didn't know how he got on at summer camp. We presumed he was fine.

But more than one parent in particular raised the point:

> I wonder how far he will be able to do these things when he leaves school. I do not have the contacts for example to enable him to pursue skiing.

I asked parents about whether they wanted to be more involved with the school than they were and whether they wanted to set up parent groups, or they thought such groups should be set up. Almost all the parents did not want to be any more involved but some would welcome more opportunity to form parents' groups, however, where they could collectively consider some of the problems they faced with their children and with the school. This was especially true in areas, fairly close to the school, where there were a group of the parents able to be in contact with one another. All of the parents welcomed visits from the school staff, which, in most instances meant visits from Eric Carbarns, the Assistant Principal Family Work.

Chapter 5

Raddery in Context

Residential special schools for children who are emotionally damaged are notoriously individualistic. I have not adopted any systematic approach in selecting other schools and communities to help me to place Raddery in a broader context. To do so would require a major research programme which has not been undertaken since 1970 when Maurice Bridgeland gave an historical and contemporary account of the special education scene for what were then called schools for 'maladjusted' children.*

In looking for background material, I have come across some other studies. These include studies undertaken by higher degree students and Inspectors' reports. There are also research studies concerned with special education generally. These provide context for visits I paid to a small number of schools and correspondence with others. A new study, funded by the Nuffield Foundation, is planned to begin in 1991, carried out by the National Children's Bureau. I understand five schools will be selected in England and that researchers will spend eight weeks studying each school and further time reviewing referral arrangements and other issues about placements. While I spent much longer than three weeks at Raddery, over a much longer period, I have only very briefly been able to get to know something about other schools. The aim, for me, therefore has been to set Raddery, as one example of 'a very special school' into

---

* BRIDGELAND, M. (1971) *Pioneering Work with Maladjusted Children*, Granada.

some kind of context. If Raddery represents a 'port' where I have harboured, I have only been able to view other places as part of a wider coastline.

There are two main purposes in trying to set Raddery in context. First, it highlights some of the distinctive features of this particular residential school and community. Secondly, it raises issues about Raddery's practice and the practice of other schools. These issues will be taken up in later chapters.

The Charterhouse Group

Raddery belongs to a loose grouping of establishments called the Charterhouse Group. They include eleven residential establishments altogether — all except Raddery being in the South, South Midlands or West of England. Many of them have a long history associated with pioneering work in special education. I visited two of these places, the Cotswold Community and New Barns.

The Cotswold Community

The main features the Cotswold Community shares with Raddery are, perhaps, the notion of the therapeutic community and the extent of individualization in pursuing a child-centred approach. Staff in both establishments will go out of their way to respond to the needs of each child, using all the skills that they possess, however unconventional or surprising the consequences. I did not, as it happened, find anything equivalent to The Oak House at The Cotswold Community, but I had the feeling I might have done.

A comparison between some of the obvious and external features of the two communities can be summarized by setting them out in columns as follows:

COMPARISON OF FEATURES OF RADDERY AND COTSWOLD COMMUNITY

	Raddery	**Cotswold**
Children		
Number	40	**50**
Age-range	Later primary or secondary	Later primary or secondary
Gender	Boys and girls	Boys only
Description	Emotionally damaged — varied backgrounds	'Unintegrated' — with background of delinquency
Location:	Rural, about three miles from village	Rural, about four miles from village
Buildings and Grounds:	Main house with attached classrooms, outbuildings, converted stables etc., including meeting room, art and science rooms and residential cottage for some children. Some staff accommodation. Hall planned. Woodland area. Animals. Also Strathallan half-way house in local community.	Core and cluster style estate, with the original core house being the administrative centre, but five separate houses, each with its own 'poly' for individualized education. Swimming pool. 300-acre farm.

Referral and Catchment Area	Education or social work authorities in the north and midland areas of Scotland, largest number from Highlands	Social services departments throughout Britain, largest number from London
Care Available:	School terms and exceptionally during part of holidays (Under review)	Up to fifty-two weeks by arrangement
Where Staff Live:	Some at Raddery others outside	All in Cotswold Community, except domestic staff and bursar
Management:	Independent company with charitable status.	Wilts CC Social Services C'tee

It is hard for me to write about the The Cotswold Community except in terms of contrast with the past. Residential special schools often owe much to the buildings and settings they inherit. I am not suggesting buildings determine practice — though they impose contraints and provide opportunities. I am suggesting there is an interaction between past and present associated with inherited buildings. Many years ago I happened to know about the Cotswold Community when it belonged to the Bruderhof or Brothers, a communitarian movement whose members escaped from Hitler to settle in rural England, and later in South America. Amongst other things, they established the farm and workshops. This was an ideal setting for an Approved School which became well known, under the charismatic leadership of C.A. Joyce (who amongst many other things, used to contribute regularly to the BBC's *Thought for the*

Day (or whatever it was called then). The school was run by the Rainer Foundation.

I visited the Cotswold School in the mid-1950s when C.A. Joyce was there. There were then three houses with regimes reflecting varying degrees of discipline. The harshest was nicknamed Belsen and a more liberal one Butlins. There was a 'quiet room' where individual recalcitrant children were locked in to meditate in front of a Quaker poster depicting two mules with the slogan 'Co-operation is better than conflict'. Mr Joyce recounted to me the pathos of a situation in his morning meeting when he asked the children to pause to think about an ex-pupil who was due to be hanged that day.

Society's ideas changed. Hanging was abolished. In due course, Approved Schools (once reformatories) became 'Community Homes'. The Rainer Foundation (after Joyce had retired) realized Cotswold had to change. Just how, using what was called a 'gulp strategy' is described graphically in one of David Wills's books: *Spare the Child*.* Its new head was another charismatic leader, Richard Balbernie. He, in turn, retired and the current Principal, whom I met on my last visit, is John Whitwell.

I found John Whitwell to be quietly spoken and clear about what he stood for. I also spoke to the Head of Education, Peter Millar. The community has some basic ideas which differ from Raddery's. 'Community' in the Cotswold sense does not really mean a single group of children. There is no common morning meeting or assembly, no regular community meeting for the whole school, no shared schooling. Contacts between children in each of the five houses are, on the one hand on rare festive occasions and, on the other, informal acquaintance in work or play on the large estate. But each of the five households operates like a mini-therapeutic community, so that group meetings and other therapeutic experiences occur within each household. There are also total community meetings for staff and John Whitwell told me that much time was spent 'working on our shared treatment philosophy'.

This 'philosophy' is the outcome of decades of experience, starting with Winnicott and Dockar-Drysdale in the 1940s and

* WILLS, W.D. (1971) *Spare the Child*, Harmondsworth, Penguin.

1950s and Balbernie's research in the 1950s and 1960s, which led to his book *Residential Work with Children.***

The features of the Cotswold Community are to be understood in terms of the strict definition of the boys who come, and therefore of their specialized needs. All the children are described, at least when they are referred, as 'unintegrated'.

In defining the meaning of 'integration' and an 'unintegrated child', John Whitwell explained that most children develop a sense of their own identity through childhood. Their egos become integrated through the security of relationships with parents and others. Many disturbed children achieve some degree of integration. But a few of those (who often present symptoms of persistent delinquency) for whom Cotswold particularly caters, are 'frozen', because of early traumatic experiences, at a primitive stage when their egos are totally unintegrated. In other words, there is no recognizable ego on which to base normal care or education. The practice at Cotswold is therefore based on allowing controlled emotional regression to undertake healing and caring at that primitive stage. This is accomplished in small numbers where individual expression is allowed with individual attention from adults. This explained the five separate houses and the five separate small 'polys' attached to them.

I visited one of the houses and, all too briefly (for they were just finishing a session) its associated poly.

The Cotswold Community today does not exhibit the Quaker donkeys pulling in opposite directions. (That, perhaps, requires quite an integrated ego to follow!) But I did find exhibited, in the house I visited, as well as in the Cotswold's prospectus a handwritten statement entitled: 'Principles by which we try to live in the households of the Cotswold Community'. It reads:

** Barbara Docker-Drysdale has for many years been involved with another Charterhouse School, the Mulberry Bush, near Oxford. She is currently a consultant to the Cotswold Community and has heavily influenced its understanding of children's needs. Her influence, of course, has been much wider.

Barbara Docker-Drysdale's latest book is called *The Provision of Primary experience: Winnicottian Work with Children and Adolescents*, London, Free Association Books, 1980.

This is our house and we value it.

It is a dreadful thing for a grown-up to hit a boy.

It is just as dreadful for a boy to hit a grown up, or another boy.

It is important to be given the chance to put things right.

There is nothing which cannot be said — in the right place, at the right time.

It is important to listen to what other people have to say.

When people are violent it is because they are not talking to other people.

There must always be food if someone is hungry.

It is important to feel clean and tidy, and cared for.

If you feel ill, tell somebody at once.

You cannot like other people if you do not like yourself.

Everyone needs to be able to trust.

It is important to be able to cry.

The truth helps.

If you give orders — grown ups or children — these must have a reason.

Anger must be understood, and put into words.

It is important to accept being in the wrong.

Scrrow must find comfort, pain must find relief, sadness must be felt.

If there are needs these must be met somehow.

Some people cannot be taught, but they can learn.

Do not be afraid to ask anything.

Some things are private.

I did actually witness a member of staff in quite a dramatic way put into practice an alternative to hitting a child at mealtime. It seemed to me at first that he was about to lay in to him in a way I have seen at some other residential establishments, but then I noticed he was more holding him, almost smothering him for a few moments.

John Whitwell later told me that 'holding only occurs as a last resort — it is in the main holding through a relationship'. However, an article he wrote in the International Journal of Therapeutic Communities also provides a possible explanation of what I witnessed:

Nothing is more difficult than to treat panic in the middle of a normally functioning group — at a mealtime, or in class, or playgroup, for example.

Earlier in the article he explains how unintegrated children cannot cope with panic in the way integrated children can:

Anyone can panic for brief periods every so often, but unintegrated children panic constantly when emotionally they are in a gap within themselves. Panic can appear as rage, fright or despair: it can result in violent acting out or total immobilization; explosion or implosion. The therapeutic treatment of panic involves holding, or containment, and very intensive care from a deeply involved therapist.

These comments are in the context of John Whitwell's argument that unintegrated children have to be treated separately from integrated children. This is the *raison d'etre* for everything that goes on at Cotswold.

To return to the meal-table. I was impressed that the staff member was controlled in his every action. Shortly after his encounter with the child at mealtime, the adult was laughing about wasps with another child and, a little later, he was zooming around the dining room with him pretending to be scared of a wasp!

There was a short meeting in the sitting room after lunch to decide who was doing the washing-up. It ended up that we all were, to the accompaniment of musical instruments augmented with saucepan lids etc. apparently in preparation for an end-of-term event.

Another short meeting in the sitting room, and various things about the afternoon arrangements were sorted out — including one boy being volunteered to show me around.

I was most impressed — even amazed — by the children's bedrooms. I have not before seen individualization taken to the point of each child designing the shape of his own bed. Most were like wooden boxes, perhaps offering greater primitive security. Later, I was to find the same principle applied to individualized places at the poly — Cotswold's alternative to school.

The poly which I saw was situated in a long attic. Children, with much coaxing, were finishing a variety of individual activities, and jumping in and out of a Wendy House. The teacher explained that normal teaching methods would be inappropriate for these children. He also told me that moving from one session to another was always difficult and time-consuming. We were on our way to swimming. With emotionally damaged — even unintegrated and frozen — children, the swimming pool is the great equalizer, just as it is for profoundly handicapped children. With such perfect strokes, who could imagine they were 'unintegrated'?

This brings me to another point John Whitwell made. Emotionally unintegrated as the children were, they were still having to cope with the feelings and the chemistry of adolescence. This was, in his view, the reason for making Cotswold a boys only place. The children had the opportunity to relate to staff of both sexes, including volunteers, like a psychology student who was also accompanying us to watch the boys swimming.

The polys provide primary and secondary education. The Head of Education told me they are considering a new venture, an alternative 'small school' for secondary children to serve the whole school, along the lines of 'small schools' developed elsewhere as alternatives to traditional education. An advantage, it was explained, for the Cotswold Community, would be that more staff could participate, drawing on the fullness of their skills backgrounds (as they are able to do at Raddery) such as playing unusual instruments, craftwork and so on.

I have not, of course, adequately described The Cotswold Community. How could I after one day spent there? In particular, I could not study during so short a visit the application of specific treatment plans for individual children. But I have seen enough to highlight the main differences from, and some similarities with, Raddery. It is fair to say that the experience and philosophy of the Cotswold Community, and of its consultant Barbara Docker-Drysdale, have considerably influenced Raddery during the past few years. This has occurred partly through visits from Raddery staff and partly through Raddery's own consultants who, in turn, have been influenced by the Cotswold philosophy.

New Barns School

New Barns School was started in 1965 by John Cross and the Homer Lane Trust. As these names suggest, there are important historical connections. The title 'New Barns' comes from the original Barns Hostel School in Scotland in the 1940s and early 1950s, pioneered by David Wills. His name and his work partly inspired by a yet earlier pioneer, Homer Lane, takes us right back to the origins of modern residential schools for emotionally damaged children in Britain. The original 'Barns Experiment' (at Peebles) was started as a means of coping with evacuees during the war who were so unruly that they could not be billetted.

Again, I have some first-hand experiences of New Barns's inheritance. As an undergraduate at Cambridge, intending at that time to become a journalist, I was persuaded to volunteer to help at a local boy's hostel called Winston House. I think my main motive was to run a model railway there! But through the influence of my mother, who was President of the Quaker-run Bedford Institute Association in East London, and having been subjected to groups of adolescents from 'the slums' descending upon our large suburban garden and adjoining woods and countryside during the war, I had more than a passing interest in the boys of Winston House and how they were treated. Intuitively, I felt something was not as it should be. The staff were kind but, to my way of thinking, lacking in any imagination.

So, as a budding journalist, I set off during a summer vacation (1950) to find out more. I visited many places in England, Ireland and Scotland. A Glasgow remand home was not to be forgotten. Because of lack of staff, boys were held for three-quarters of an hour in an imposed most un-Quakerly silence. The buildings were cramped and appalling. Then I went to Rossie Farm School near Arbroath. Here were new imposing buildings with all the space one could wish for and a new head proud of what he was doing. But it was regimented.

At last a Quaker at Edinburgh said to me 'Have you heard of Barns?' I hadn't. It was some forty miles to the south of Edinburgh near Jedburgh.

Having visited hundreds of establishments in my time, I

have learnt the significance of how the visitor is welcomed. Two ten-year old boys met me off my bus and, to my amazement, one of them took me by the hand. He led me up a long track to an old stately home (now demolished). After a brief discussion with the then head, Ben Stoddard, I was thrown into the throng of community, full of noise and excitement.

For the first time, I felt I was with people who knew what they were doing and why they were doing it. The experience was the first nudge to postpone my journalistic career in favour of some kind of work like this. Its influence was to make me feel I had to be involved.

The principles on which Barns was based, practised by Ben Stoddard and his staff and written about by David Wills* who had earlier started the school as Barns Hostel near Peebles, reached the deepest aspects of human behaviour and human experience and applied these to the tasks in hand — namely the care and re-education of children who were at once deprived of a normal family life and uncontrollable in ordinary schools. In two sentences, it seemd to me it was, firstly love in action, the kind of love I knew about from my own much more fortunate (though by no means always idyllic) Christian upbringing. Secondly, it was a statement that in this work of love there can be no compromises. Only the best is good enough.

I returned to Barns as a student helper during the subsequent Christmas vacation (in deep snow!) and the following summer I paid my first visit to Bodenham Manor School, amidst the apple orchards near Hereford. This was where David Wills was then practising. Bodenham was seen by David Wills as an advance on Barns for several reasons. It was co-educational. The care and the educational aspects were in harmony, since David Wills (himself a social worker) was clearly in charge. The head teacher at that time was Howard Jones — to become a well-known sociologist and criminologist. One of the assistant teachers was John Cross.

By the following year, I was completing a postgraduate course in social administration involving practical work

---

* WILLS, D.W. (1949) *The Barns Experiment*, London, Allen and Unwin.

placements. I managed to persuade my tutor to send me to Bodenham Manor and the placement was extended on a paid basis. So for many years afterwards — in fact until after I had become involved with Raddery — Bodenham (or perhaps I should say David Wills) was the embodiment for me of what seemed good practice in residential work with children.

John Cross must have been affected more deeply than I was — or at least in a different way. I felt that good though Bodenham was, alternative work could be undertaken to prevent children having to leave their homes in the first place. For the next nine years I worked with Family Service Units, which offered intensive whole-family support mostly in inner-city areas. It did not always succeed! I learnt that however much family support is offered (and it should be offered) some children need an alternative therapeutic environment.

Meanwhile, John Cross, together with a number of others, had found the support they needed to form the Homer Lane Trust and to start New Barns, in a no-less beautiful rural setting, in a village called Toddington, miles from anywhere (Cheltenham being the nearest town) on the borders of Gloucestershire and Worcestershire. I had visited, I think, twice before in its early days, before returning recently to update my experiences for the specific purposes of this book.

The historical experiences I have shared help to explain some of the most remarkable features of New Barns. Twenty eight children (it used to be thirty plus) share community life with about 18 adults for six term-time periods of six weeks each during the year. For the remaining six shorter holiday periods, they return to their parents or other carers.

John explained to me: 'It is not a place where the children are resident and the staff are not resident but only on duty'. When later I asked how much time staff had 'off', I was soon made to realize I had asked a silly question and that I should have known better!

'Off what?' John asked me in return. 'Adults' (not staff, for they are not appointed to specific staff appointments at all, but come with their varied backgrounds and qualifications to join the community as caring adults), I was told, have one-and-half days a week (during term periods) of free time — free that is from specific functions or duties. There is no shift system (which certainly makes for simplicity in organizational terms!). When staff are 'free' they are still, if they choose to be on the premises, 'with the children'.

New Barns is described as being mainly a 'middle school' for children aged 7 to 13+, but now concentrates on primary ages. As at Raddery, changes reflect the increasingly difficult children now being referred. The responses have been, in a sense, opposite. Raddery has expanded and become more complex with different 'venues' for different groups of children. New Barns has slightly contracted in numbers as well as in age-range. (John explained that economic factors had entered into the decision to take more than twenty-eight children in the past but that they would not take more now in the interests of sustaining what is considered the optimum viable size for the community.)

John showed me around the school, with many extensions (built mainly by the community themselves) since my previous visits. The buildings are in two main complexes. This, John explained, was for architectual rather than policy reasons. The main complex comprises the original old house, used for living accommodation including kitchen and dining room, with extensions to new classrooms, a hall and other rooms. The second complex, just a few yards away, mainly comprises additional living accommodation.

Living accommodation includes interspersed bedrooms for adults and for children — usually two or three children together (as at Raddery). But at Raddery there are no staff resident in the same building — staff houses are in separate buildings from where the children sleep, except for staff on evening or night duty. At New Barns there is no 'night' duty in that sense. Adults are simply present in adjacement rooms when the children have gone to bed.

Of course, adults at New Barns do have, against this background of their primary role as adult members of the community, specific roles and responsibilities (as distinct from fixed posts). Whilst everybody shares in almost everything, some people do more cooking, some people do more teaching, some people provide a focus for what, in some establishments, would be seen as 'care' responsibilities. Furthermore, as John explained to me, somebody with a teaching qualification would tend to have a specific teaching responsibility. There is, however, no absolute requirement to match formal qualifications with functions. Teaching, for example, (in classes of 5–6 as at Raddery) can be shared amongst a wider range of adults than would otherwise be the case.

Much of what goes on in terms of the interaction between adults and children would be familiar and acceptable to a visitor from Raddery. Individual relationships are all-important. They are relationships based on understanding and love. Perhaps adults at New Barns are more informally affectionate in physical terms than at Raddery (though affection is important at Raddery too as the studies of children in Chapter 4 testified). John himself addresses children as 'love' or 'dear' and, to the children (and adults) he is 'John'. At Raddery children would tend to say 'Mr Dean'. These differences are not in themselves necessarily important. They may reflect two basic differences:

1   Raddery has mainly older children.
2   Raddery children usually maintain contact with their families during term-time, going home every third week-end or sometimes more often. New Barns operates with four longer term-time periods. As a brochure for parents states:

> The regular pattern of terms and holidays maintains vital links with home, diminishes the possibility of the child being excluded by the family, prevents too comfortable an adaptation to residential life, and keeps alive the issues and conflicts, the painful realities and the positive motivations which are the material for our work with the child.

In other words, New Barns can be said to offer an alternative to the child's home for shorter term-time periods. It aims to be like a good home in the sense that it provides the kind of affection and informality one would expect in a good home. John feels that the experience and work that take place within the community and the home must not be confused. While there are regular meetings between the parents and New Barns, together with someone from the referring agency, parents are not especially encouraged to visit, though they can if they wish (and can get there). There is no accommodation for them to stay the night at school. John explained that to a large extent, New Barns was intensive, self-contained and 'exclusive'.

'Exclusive' is a term used to describe a foster or adoption placement which excludes contact with the natural parents. An inclusive placement aims to include such contacts. While borrowing the foster-care term, John emphasized New Barns was not in any sense offering an alternative to home, quite the contrary. The overall aim was to return children to their normal families, and to normal secondary schools after their period of about four years was completed at New Barns. He stated that about 75 per cent of children did return to ordinary schools.

Work with families is conducted mainly by local authority social service departments, based on reviews between the school, social workers and others including the parents.

As at Raddery, New Barns aims to accept children presenting a range of emotional and behavioural difficulties. Some are described in terms of Docker-Drysdale's term 'unintegrated'. But here John made an important caveat (which I must say I personally found helpful). He said such children often had 'pockets of good experience which you can respond to'. 'Unintegrated' provided a conceptual framework for greater understanding of children's behaviour and their needs. This was not the same thing as labelling children themselves as 'unintegrated' as though that was all there was to them. This must also be helpful, surely, in understanding the needs of Warren and of David whom we considered in Chapter 4.

I felt that at New Barns, adults would have to be extraordinarily integrated, for where can they turn to outside for daily support?

I was heartened to learn that staff do, on average, stay for longer than the children and some have been at the school for the twenty-five years since it started. They cannot, however, have families of their own. John explained there would not be accommodation within the community and that to make such accommodation and to welcome staff children would distract from the work of the community. So all of the staff are either single people or childless couples. Their lives are devoted to the children. But they do get respite during holiday periods, though even then part of each holiday is devoted (as at Raddery) to reviews and planning.

As at Raddery, the spiritual values underpinning the school are recognized, though in different ways. Each day begins at New Barns with a short period when the community gathers in silence. The Quaker influence is common to Raddery's morning meeting — John Cross himself being a Quaker (as Wills was).

Shared responsibility also takes similar forms, only that at New Barns meetings are held after each mealtime. I had remembered community meeting at New Barns as more confrontory than at Raddery, where there is more emphasis on consensus and harmony. I had recalled for John an occasion when he had 'gone to town' and really shouted at a boy who had insulted another child on racial grounds. John said this was perhaps a good example of when confrontation might have been used, but confrontation was useless, indeed potentially damaging unless it reached down to some real values, understanding and insight within the child. Perhaps more important in community meetings were the processes that led to resolution, reparation and the gaining of insights.

In any event, he said there was less confrontation in community meetings now than there might have been once, partly because children were younger and partly because they were certainly initially more emotionally fragmented and fragile, which would make confrontation irrelevant and inappropriate.

This did not mean, however, that New Barns was moving away from shared responsibility.

Classroom teaching was possibly about mid-way between Raddery's holistic (but still, in some ways, fairly formal) classroom teaching and Cotswold's abandonment of teaching (at least at primary level) in their 'polys'. The teaching I witnessed during my very cursory visit to New Barns was mainly adults sharing educational experience with children, usually with an arm round them. One child was sitting by himself not wanting to participate. It was more like education in an alternative home setting than a school. John elaborated on one aspect I could see for myself. Every moment of the day was potentially educational. During lunch an adult was possibly giving the most formal teaching lesson he ever did, arising naturally from children's conversations.

John explained to me that New Barns is sometimes questioned because people get the impression, because of the apparent low-key nature of both educational and therapeutic 'programmes', that theoretical perspectives to understanding behaviour and needs are overlooked. John said that on the contrary, such perspectives and insights were at the heart of their work, being used in a total understanding of children's needs and in responding in a total way.

Such an approach suggests an enormous, and perhaps quiet, confidence most of the adults must have in what they know about and in what they are doing.

Other Schools

So far, I have set Raddery in the context of two schools which belong to the Charterhouse Group. What of the much larger number of special schools for emotionally damaged children outside this exclusive group and what about work with emotionally damaged children in special units often alongside children with other kinds of special needs? What about arrangements where disturbed children are supported in ordinary classes?

In 1989 the Department of Education and Science published a survey of 'pupils with emotional/behavioural difficulties in maintained special schools and units' in England and Wales. Fifty-seven schools and nine units were selected — quite a large number, although the report recognizes 'within the limits of the exercise it was not possible to ensure a representative sample of institutions from all areas of the country'.

The report makes, on the whole, depressing reading. For example:

In the residential schools a satisfactory level of child care staff was found in 60 per cent of cases but the hostel attached to one of the units was not staffed adequately. It is clearly a matter for concern that child care staffing levels were unsatisfactory in so many instances. The quality of care and supervision was adversely affected by this shortfall in some schools. (*Paragraph 34*)

In only a few schools were the organizational arrangements fully satisfactory. Their effectiveness derived from a well-defined and accepted view of the school's task in relation to its pupils and their special educational needs, reflected in clearly articulated curricular aims and objectives. For the most part such coherence and cohesion were absent. (*Paragraph 40*)

Very seldom was the school responsive to the needs of the tiny minority of girls. (*Paragraph 41*)

The many lessons disrupted by poor attitudes and uncontrolled behaviour were frequently also characterized by inappropriate teaching styles and stereotyped approaches to learning on the part of the teachers. Ill-judged content of work, poor match of tasks to pupils' capabilities and lack of pace were also frequently noted. Very seldom was there any evidence in the work seen in classrooms or in pupil's exercise or workbooks of planned progression or continuity of educational experience. (*Paragraph 52*)

In only a very few instances was there a clearly stated school policy on assessment and record keeping. (*Paragraph 54*)

At the same time, the report noted that 'every school subscribed to the view that pupils with emotional/behavioural difficulties need security, need opportunity to build affective relationships with adults and peers and need to learn new and more affective appropriate modes of behaviour' (*Paragraph 61*).

The quality of relationships in the schools was often good, but seldom appeared to be used as a base from which to initiate and support changes in behaviour or attitudes in any planned or systematic way. (*Paragraph 62*)

However, the report also reports 'considerable evidence of successful practice' in schools which were 'places of great warmth, vitality and strength'. It goes on to say:

It is not surprising that, for the most part, the residential schools were the more successful in this regard. (*Paragraph 63*)

A more limited Scottish study makes similar broad criticisms.*

East Quinton School, East Sussex

One of the schools I corresponded with was East Quinton School at Bexhill-on-Sea. They were not included in the DEA survey but the headteacher, Jon Fogell, referred to the report in his letter to me. He wrote:

It is fair to say that a year ago this school represented many of the observations that were made (in the report).

However, he claimed that since then 'It is my belief that the style of provision being worked towards at East Quinton School forms a model of residential education which will equip it for the demands of the twenty-first century'.

East Quinton is a day and boarding school maintained by East Sussex County Council. It caters for forty boarding boys, fifteen boarding girls (in an annexe) and ten day pupils. A leaflet intended, amongst others, for parents lists six aims of the school. The central educational aim is 'the same for all pupils in

* SCOTTISH OFFICE (SED) (1990) *Choosing With Care*. A Report of HM Inspectors of Schools on the provision for pupils with behavioural, emotional and social difficulties.

all schools', namely, that the child 'should develop as an individual contributory member of society'. The other aims include to develop 'qualities of integrity and perseverance under difficulties'; to provide a coherent framework to develop 'thorough knowledge, concepts, skills and attitudes'; to enable children to 'understand their own problems and find acceptable ways of coping with them'; 'to enable parents and children to improve their understanding of each other' and, lastly, 'to return the pupil to as normal a school and social environment as possible, as soon as possible'.

Resident children maintain contact with home during term-time as well as in holidays. The school is open two out of three term-time week-ends. Children attend on a five-day week basis at an 'appropriate time' and the aim is that all final year pupils will attend on a day basis, though depending on home circumstances.

The school is an all-through one, but divided into Bands, Junior, Senior and Leavers. There is evidence of planning at each stage appropriate for the age-group whilst following the National Curriculum. The primary stage features a broad approach (including music, drama, practical and artistic skills and physical education) and teaching is based on individual children's needs with a 'minimum of movement between teachers'.

In contrast, the secondary band tries 'to maintain a style which is similar to mainstream secondary schools', with added emphasis on vocational educational support, personal and social education, while 'basic education in English and Mathematics is general to each pupil's individual needs'. Some teaching is provided through links with mainstream schools.

The final year at school is in the Leavers Band. All pupils take part in a work experience scheme. 'At present pupils spend one day each week in the workplace and much of the subsequent work in the classroom is based on their experiences at work'.

Out of school activities, especially week-ends when children are there, are broadly based depending on staff and children's interests. Children are encouraged to join local clubs and other activities in the community.

Each resident pupil at the school has a child care officer, a class teacher and a personal tutor. They each have a daily log book which monitors their behaviour throughout each day. Behaviour is then discussed at daily school meetings and weekly group meetings. Emphasis is placed on rewarding good behaviour through a merit system which gives pupils letters to take home for praiseworthy behaviour. The school aims to share with pupils 'our desire for an orderly and compassionate community'. Work with families and links between external agencies is co-ordinated through the school's teacher/counsellor.

Swalcliffe Park School

This is another school I corresponded with. It is, like Raddery, run by an independent charitable trust. The school was established in 1965 with grants from the Nuffield Provincial Hospital Trust with assistance from the Department of Education and Science.

Situated six miles from Banbury in rural Oxfordshire, Swalcliffe Park accommodates fifty pupils (boys only) of secondary age and a limited number of day pupils with 'a wide range of learning, emotional and behavioural difficulties'. Based on a four-term year, it maintains close links with families both in term-time and during holiday periods.

The school has a high investment in teachers and modern classrooms to cater for the educational needs of what appears to be a diverse group of children. A remedial department caters for children needing intensive assistance in basic skills. For older children, there are close links with the local College of Further Education as well as work experience placements.

Like Raddery, the school has a number of 'houses' (what Raddery would call 'venues') to meet different kinds of needs. East House acts 'mainly as a reception for boys who lack motivation and self-discipline and require a high level of supervision'. The unit is highly structured and free time is organized by the staff.

West House is for boys who are 'generally more responsive and need help to acquire social and life skills that will enable them to develop as individuals'. Boys are held more accountable for their actions 'so that they can be made aware of the decision-making process'.

Attic House provides an environment for greater self-discipline and self-evaluation. Boys are encouraged also to participate in a wider range of experiences to help their self-awareness and confidence.

Finally, for post-16 boys, George House (purpose-built within the school's twenty-acre grounds) is 'completely independent from the main school' and has different kinds of accommodation to cater either for independent bed-sits or small group living. It encourages 'a high level of independence' with all boys following an individual work experience programme 'allowing them to draw up a personal set of criteria to use at a later date when seeking full-time employment'.

A separate and prominent section in the school's brochure is headed 'Future'. It points out that the school is constantly developing. Current developments include a small 'independent flat' for use in the main house. Flexibility is stressed 'both in buildings and staff structure'.

Boys' reviews are held annually with parents and reports prepared every six months.

The range of outdoor activities is, like Raddery's, impressive, including sailing and canoeing. Boys are encouraged to join the Youth Hostels Association (YHA).

Swalcliffe is already well staffed and equipped but is 'committed to increase staff levels and a range of professional support'. The latter already includes the part-time services of a psychologist and a psychiatrist. The principal, Maurice Cooling, is very alive to current issues in the education and care of the range of children he is responsible for and has himself undertaken research in this field. He is currently undertaking what he describes as 'a small piece of work relating to pupil perceptives of their residential experiences'.

In correspondence to check the accuracy of this description, Maurice Cooling gave me some further information about the school's history. It was Richard Balbernie who started the original Swalcliffe Park School (out of which the present school developed) before he moved to Cotswold. After reading my draft of this chapter, Maurice Cooling commented 'One is constantly reminded of how inter-connected places become with their personnel'.

Linnwood Hall School

Schools can change very quickly. One school which has changed dramatically and which David Dean suggested I should visit, is Linnwood Hall in Fife, Scotland. The Head, Dr John Tollan, told me that before he came two years ago, the school offered long-term education and care. Now it provides short-time residential or day support and is 'evolving towards an educative community in which young people and their families can work through those problems requiring day or residential placement towards the aim of re-integration to home, community and, where appropriate, school or work'.

As I talked with John Tollan, I soon realized he was in the 'top league' of unusually talented people associated with special education in this field. Lively, but relaxed, he looked hardly old enough to have acquired the breadth of experience and qualifications that he has. He has taught in a variety of schools and at teacher training college. He has triple professional qualifications as teacher, social worker and educational psychologist. His approach is eclectic in making his school a 'centre for excellence'.

In many respects, the contrast with Raddery could not be greater. Linnwood Hall, for children aged 11–16, is situated not in the country but on a twelve-acre site (once a convalescent home for miners) in Leven surrounded by housing in an Educational Priority Area. Although Fife has some very pleasant countryside, population-wise it is an industrial area with a strong local authority commitment to education. Linwood Hall is one of five local special schools for children with 'complex social, emotional and behavioural difficulties'.

In this context, Linnwood Hall can specialize. It does not aim to take, for example, children who are primarily delinquent. Nor does it take children who could be better placed at a well-known adolescent psychiatric unit, Playfield House, attached to Stratheden Psychiatric Hospital near Cupar. As what one might call a minimal function, it aims to receive children from ordinary schools, assess, understand and respond to the full range of educational and emotional problems and needs presented, and return them to ordinary schools as soon as possible with all the necessary support. But more than this, the school aims to try to prevent children coming in the first place. This task is approached in a number of ways. A small unit has been set up away from the main school where children from ordinary schools can attend part-time on a day basis. The school also operates a variety of outreach programmes to support staff and children in ordinary schools. In various ways, the school is involved in the local community and the local community in the school.

John Tollan stressed the importance of tackling attitudes in schools and in the community. It was sometimes hard for ordinary schools to accept children back, after they had been referred to Linnwood Hall. It was easy for schools to see the referral to a special school as a 'disposal', not only of the child but of the problem. Another theme I picked up from talking to John Tollan was his commitment to collaboration between services. For example, he told me of plans to transfer the adolescent psychiatric unit to Linnwood Hall in a proposed joint venture between the local authority Education Department (which runs Linnwood Hall) and the Health Board. This multi-disciplinary initiative would be designed to create an integrated 'centre of excellence' catering for a wider range of young people with complex emotional and behavioural difficulties.

Linnwood Hall has most in common with Raddery in terms of a holistic approach to education and to informal teaching methods, which has been recognized through the presentation to the school of a national curriculum award. Several 'classrooms' I visited at Linnwood Hall were like homely sitting rooms in an old Victorian house, although the school was not lacking in equipment. Bedrooms were fairly normal too (and in this respect more like Raddery's than Cotswold's highly individualized bedrooms). But many children only stay at Linnwood Hall part of the week. A lad showing me around pointed out the room he shared with another boy — but each of them only stays one night a week as part of a phased weaning process from initial full-time residence.

As at Raddery, and traditionally at some other schools, children are involved in the school's continued programme of building development. One of the results of this, I was told, was the absence of vandalism from within the school. Perhaps the involvement with the local community also prevents vandalism from outside.

Linnwood Hall has more sophisticated assessment procedures than, as yet, operate at Raddery. Assessment at Linnwood leads to action and it is the wide horizons of such action that impressed me — extending to parents as well as teachers in ordinary schools and, through other services, to an ever-broader 'educative community'. Within this scheme, there are two key staff roles, one called the 'mentor' and the other the 'key worker'. The mentor role of 'individual educational programme management', along with teaching specific areas of the curriculum, combines teaching with pastoral care, collaboration with other staff and colleagues elsewhere, communication with parents and outreach with other educational settings. The 'key worker' role of care management incorporates parenting and professional caring, and also collaboration with other staff and colleagues and communicating with parents.

The ultimate goal of Linnwood Hall might be to make itself redundant as a residential special school — though not as a multi-disciplinary resource centre committed to supporting children and their families, both from and in local schools. However, in the meantime, as at Raddery, attention is being given to the needs of more disturbed children who are 'emotionally stuck' and a new interdependence unit is planned within the school for post-16 children to promote their integration into the community.

Perth External Behavioural Support System

There are many different approaches to preventing the need for some children to attend long-term special schools. To find out more about just one example in my own home locality I contacted one of the educational psychologists in Perth, Peter Kaye. He told me about what is called the 'External Behaviour Support System' for secondary school children. A team of teachers is available under a co-ordinator. A variety of support options include support within the ordinary school, withdrawal from ordinary class, work experience, Duke of Edinburgh Award Scheme, home tuition, college or link courses and individual tuition activities (or combinations of these).

Meanwhile, a day unit in Perth for children with behavioural problems had closed. This was partly because children who were referred were presenting increasingly complex difficulties, partly because children were in danger of losing out educationally in a small separate unit and partly because the increased number of disruptive children could not be handled. The school had previously aimed at a balance between 'troubled and troublesome'. It was interesting, therefore, to learn that the External Behavioural Support System (EBSS) had come into being to support children in ordinary schools where separate special provision could not cope so well, bearing in mind the EBSS deals with children on an individual basis and does not offer 'groupwork'.

Peter Kaye explained it was too soon to evaluate the new system but he did give me some figures about its usage in Perth. Of forty-two children referred, twenty-eight had been accepted. Fifteen of these had been dealt with through an individual programme combining off-site and in-school components. Seven had been dealt with entirely off-site and eight exclusively in their ordinary school.

In relating such schemes to the Raddery experience, one is faced with the difficulty of not knowing to what extent the children are comparable. Peter Kaye suggested that children who needed to attend a residential setting like Raddery would not be likely to be included in the Perth external behavioural support system.

Leningrad Special School

Finally, I want to give at least a flavour of placing Raddery in an international context. The obvious example to choose is the Leningrad Special School which both children and staff from Raddery visited on an exchange basis (See Chapters 2 and 3).

In a report on his first visit to the Leningrad school, David Dean first said something about the context of special education in Russia (November, 1989). He quoted Professor Vladimir Lubovski, Director of the Research Institute for Defectology of the Academy of Pedagogic Sciences of the USSR:

> Special Education is an organic part of the public edu-
> cation system and has exactly the same tasks as the
> normal school. It creates the most favourable conditions
> for the correctional education that are applied throughout
> the educational process.

These 'conditions' include an emphasis on shared responsibility or 'self-government', amongst children to help one another, an emphasis on work, and promoting a philosophy of good Soviet citizenship (1989). Special schools are separate from ordinary schools. The shared responsibility is exercized within the special system, and within specialist schools within that system. However, there are proportionately fewer children in special schools in Russia than in Britain, with more emphasis traditionally on ordinary schools coping, with support, with children having what we would term mild learning difficulties or simple rather than complex special needs.

The Leningrad school is one of 150 special schools for children with behavioural difficulties. It has 270 boys, aged 11–16, and 107 staff — very large by British standards. (Children who are disturbed but who have not committed offences would be expected to be coped with within ordinary schools, with support, for example, from parents' employers, and sometimes the police.) The school is broken down into smaller groups insofar as class-groups of twenty also share the same dormitory accommodation. There is also a house system, largely to promote competition.

The school is one of five which especially draw their inspiration from the Russian educational pioneer, Anton Makarenko. His ideas, based on practical educational experiments with adolescent delinquent boys, featured in the brief flowering period for new ideas after the Revolution and before Stalin clamped down.

Makarenko himself had some protection as the protege of

Lenin's wife. His ideas, incidentally, were influential in the West as well as in Russia and one can trace direct links between the shared responsibility philosophy and practice of Makarenko in his book *Road to Life** and Homer Lane, David Wills and others. (Wills, however, did not always share Makarenko's enthusiasm for re-education through participation in hard physical work, though this idea, too, was widely shared internationally in the 1920s and later.)

Shared responsibility and an emphasis on work featured at the Leningrad school.

Shared responsibility is based on a meritocracy. The main decision-making body, an 'Activities Council' comprised an elected group of seventeen boys with seven reservists and was steered by the Principal, Yuri Nepomnashi, and the Director of Studies. David Dean commented after his visit: 'One wonders what feelings are experienced by those who are not elected'. There was also an Academic Board, chaired by a boy, which decided upon and monitored aspects of the education pro-gramme. David Dean gave an example of how it operated:

> Recently, the school was offered the opportunity to continue following the full curriculum common to day schools throughout the country not to have to submit to examinations. The boys voted to continue taking the examinations explaining to me that they would need to go on to vocational or technical schools afterwards. Listening to them explaining how this decision was taken left me in no doubt that there was more than a trace of appropriate pride in the outcome and, as one who is highly critical of the whole business of examining and proscribing from the results, I could not deny the self-esteem gained by the achievers.

David Dean added that the numbers of lessons of forty-five minutes allocated to each subject in the curriculum matched ordinary schools with two lessons a week added in most in-stances. Physical training amounted to four hours a week.

* MAKARENKO, A.A. (1974) *Road to Life*, Central Books.

Of classroom methods, David Dean commented that teaching was 'formal, collective and subdued'. (One wonders how far Makarenko would have approved?) David Dean had the blow softened for him:

> Had I not given a lecture to mature students in one of Leningrad's higher institutes the night before, I might have wondered at the sight of pupils standing up to answer questions put by the teacher. Like the uniform which is common to all Soviet pupils under fifteen years of age, the habit of rising to one's feet to answer questions is universal throughout educational establishments.

The second main feature of the Leningrad school was the importance of the work-place, including manufacturing workshops and a cafe. The Director of the cafe, aged 14, was elected by his comrades. The workshops, in which each boy spent two and a half hours a day, with twenty-six staff, earned 300,000 roubles a year from items they produced and marketed.

The workshop staff were men and David Dean commented that they and the 'regime men who undertook live night duty and generally patrol the buildings made up almost the whole male presence'. As in many British special schools (but not at Raddery) there was a preponderance of women amongst the seventeen teachers. A paediatrician attended regularly and a psychiatrist came daily. There was no psychologist, but David Dean said the school regretted this. As, perhaps, in every country, there is a scepticism about the role of more academic consultants. The Principal was quoted as saying: 'Too often they don't understand their task: they write their theses!'

* * *

How can we summarize these many different approaches to the education, care and treatment of children with 'very special needs', as we called them at the start of the book?

Leaving aside, for the moment, what must be examples of bad practice, by any reasonable standard, referred to in the DES Report of 1989, most or all of the schools I have visited, revisited, or simply read about or corresponded with, have several things in common.

Most of them acknowledge they are in the process of rapid change. This is largely because more difficult children are now being referred than was the case in the past. It is also, perhaps, because of greater awareness of what some other schools are doing in response to the current challenge. This challenge comes from several sources. There are those who want to see an end to special schools of any kind in favour of integration with mainstream schools. At the same time, the price of failure in terms of the scale of problems, both for children and young adults, is increasingly alarming. If schools, like those examples of good practice we have reviewed, were not there, and if ordinary schools were (and are) unable to cope with, let alone address, the problems of the children present, at what cost child abuse? At what cost the pain of a divided family? At what cost the consequences of failure for these children to join, in their despair or conflict, the ranks of the homeless, the drug addicts, the prisoners or other social outcasts or isolates? And what price for their children?

So the best schools and therapeutic communities are setting higher and broader goals for themselves in response to a wider challenge. Specifically, most of them are seeing the difficulties of responding to the needs of children who are 'emotionally stuck', whom one can only understand in terms of a lack of basic 'integration', even though there may be, as John Cross said, 'pockets of good experience which you can respond to'.

Apart from this, the over-riding impression is of the very varied starting-points different schools have, depending on their previous history, how they were started, how they have changed from their starting-points and of the interaction between personalities, often great personalities, philosophies and locations with buildings, often fine buildings and fine locations. You cannot escape from past influences specific to the establishment you work in. Some would perhaps like to. John Tollan, head of Linnwood Hall, told me he would have ideally liked to have started afresh when he came with an entirely new staff. Perhaps Balbernie would, too, when the Cotswold Approved School was transformed into the Cotswold Community. But even if they could have changed the staff overnight, it still would not have been an entirely fresh start. Wolodymyr Radysh, who is an architect with the Camphill Movement, once told me that buildings have a life of their own as their use is developed. Having seen how so many special schools have evolved with their buildings and where their buildings are placed, I know what he meant.

I have written the above after considering but rejecting various more academic comparative frameworks for the special schools we are concerned with. For example, Mike Toman, ex-depute at Raddery (who moved on to become head of Craigerne school run by Barnardos in Scotland, before it closed in the face of some of the pressures I have referred to, and who now heads a private school in Athens) told me schools might be placed along a continuum according to whether they gave greater priority to education or to therapy. While some schools may neglect one or the other of these components, it is clear from the comparisons I have made that the most ambitious establishments give equal priority to both — if indeed they can make any meaningful distinction.

Another continuum might be between isolation and integration with mainstream schools. Here again, this is largely a false distinction when one takes into account the different needs that children attending different schools have. Nobody wants to isolate children with special needs from mainstream schools for the sake of it. It may be that the worst examples of special school practice are worse than the best support schemes in ordinary schools. But for children who need an alternative living environment for at least a large amount of their time, and where ordinary schools are not able to cope with the educational or caring needs these children have, special schools will maintain the links in different ways.

The starting point for this book was that Raddery was a very special school for children with very special needs. This chapter has helped us to confirm this, but also to see that it is not the only such very special school. Just the few I have considered, out of many others I might have, show that Raddery, like other schools, has much to contribute and much to learn as a caring, educational and therapeutic community.

Part II

Policy and Practice Implications

Chapter 6

Residential Child Care

What Does Residential Child Care Mean?

Before we get further into the debate about the integration of special schools into mainstream education, I want to look more closely at the caring aspect of residential special schools. What do we mean today when we say 'residential child care'?

For a whole variety of reasons most children spend part of their lives away from their parental homes. One of my own children, aged 10, spent a week away from home this summer to attend a holiday camp. When I was aged 10, I was evacuated to a residential boarding school three hundred miles from home. Though the number is diminishing, some children in the West of Scotland live in residential hostels (or in some cases lodgings) in order to attend secondary schools.

Any child residing away from home needs 'care', as he or she does in their own home. The 'care' will not be the same as it is at home. The adults in the caring roles are not the child's parents. The child will know the difference and the carers will be sensitive to this knowledge too. They will not want to usurp the parents, but they will want to meet the child's continuing needs, which are constant in any setting, for physical and emotional security, stimulation, comfort, adventure, knowledge, friends, decision-making and responsibility, for play and, as they get older, opportunities for work.

All of this applies to children with special needs. A child

with complex learning difficulties, for example, is likely to need extra stimulation as well as all the other components of care.

A child who has been emotionally damaged needs extra security, extra comfort, extra opportunities for growth. The difference here is that sometimes, because of hurt and damage from within the family, the child can only begin to experience what he or she needs away from parents. But the parents and home still profoundly matter to the child.

All children also need understanding.

Professor Bryan Williams of Dundee University has recently argued that 'understanding people' is a neglected topic in social science and social work literature, yet surely crucial to the helping professions? * This is certainly evident when we come up against the complexity — indeed the mystery — of the behavior of children. Professor Williams argued that there were artistic as well as technical aspects of understanding people.

> There are senses in which the whole process of coming to understand another person is like trying to grasp the author's meaning when reading a novel.

There are many dimensions to understanding, but the most important, as Professor Williams points out, is that it means 'getting to know you' as well as 'knowing about you'. Children need to know that those who care for them have got to know them and that they do not merely know about them.

This applies especially to children who may feel, because of emotional damage, that they have never been understood. For the same reason, more effort may be needed to achieve such an understanding.

I have dwelt on these elementary considerations partly because they may be overlooked in the perennial arguments about who does what and which agencies do what. Domestics at Raddery are called 'houseworkers' to emphasize that they, too, are members of staff care teams. In a caring residential school, teachers will try to understand children and to meet their care needs in and out of class as much as will the care staff.

* WILLIAMS, B. (1990) *Understanding People: Art and Science in Social Work*, University of Dundee Department of Social Work Publications Service.

At the agency level, it has been policy for some years for Social Services Departments (Social Work Departments in Scotland) to try to minimize residential child care provision, especially so-called long-term children's homes. The children's needs have not necessarily changed. It is the provision that has changed. More attempts are made now to adopt or to foster. More attempts are made to support children in their own homes. In many instances there is no doubt that this is laudable.

Child Care and Education

Yet for some children who have been emotionally damaged — the children we described as having very special needs — such solutions are not, of themselves, sufficient. And if the Social Services Departments do not have the provision, the residential care needs of children are sought elsewhere — including, and perhaps especially, in residential special schools. All the evidence from all the schools I have had contact with suggests that this is what has been happening. Children who once would have gone into residential childrens homes provided by the local authorities (or sponsored by local authorities in homes run by voluntary agencies) are now finding their way into residential special schools or communities.

Is this right? Should residential special schools substitute for children's homes?

The changes in policy provide an opportunity for referring agencies to sort out more carefully whether a child needs special schooling or residential therapeutic care or (as at Raddery) both. What they are unlikely to need, however, unless perhaps in a few cases on a very short-term basis, is special schooling attached to, but not integrated with, a residential therapeutic environment.

In other words, if a school is only concerned with teaching, and any care is a kind of adjunct, there is a split which this type of child (by definition) cannot cope with. If they could cope with school, as school, they would (perhaps with support) attend an ordinary school.

So the special school with a hostel attached is not likely to be the best environment for meeting the needs of emotionally damaged children away from home. Furthermore, such schools, as the DES report quoted in Chapter 5 suggested, are often bad or indifferent even in narrow educational terms. Lack of care and understanding out of class affects what goes on in class — and vice versa.

But if a residential school can offer much more than this — and we have seen what different schools can offer — does it matter which agency provides it? In a general sense it need not matter. The Cotswold Community is managed by a Social Services Department. Linnwood Hall is managed by an Education Department. However, there may be problems for the managers to grapple with. For example, care staff tend to be devalued (in terms of salaries) compared with teachers in a school.

Child Care and Mental Health Care

Apart from the question of education, it may be asked: 'Is child care enough' — for children who are emotionally damaged?

This question is prompted because when I interviewed Melvyn Rose, of the Peper Harow Foundation, and showed him the proposed outline of chapter titles for this book, he commented that perhaps I also needed a chapter on implications for policy and practice in 'mental health'. He said there was not the conceptual framework in the social services to take into account the needs of children who suffered from 'emotional and developmental injury, as a result of psychological deprivation and psycho-developmental injury'.

Is this true? Does 'child care' not include the means to understand and respond to the child's mental health problems, as well as having a concern for his physical health and social needs? Does it include understanding about emotional damage? At the level of individual caring — the loving and understanding tasks of adults for children which I earlier summarized — it surely must do!

I said in Chapter 3 that a holistic approach to education, as interpreted at Raddery, had length, breadth and depth. These dimensions should include an understanding of any child's emotional and — where applicable — psycho-social needs. As a principle, this is inscribed in almost every piece of professional social work literature that has ever been written on the subject!

After writing that last sentence, I thought I should put it to the test! I reached to the shelf of books next to me and picked out the first one with any relevance to this topic. It is the book *Adoption and Fostering: Why and How* by Carole R. Smith, and produced by the British Association of Social Workers. Turning to page 37, I found the following:

> The factors which influence individual development are complex and as we all know some children will come through appalling experiences relatively unscathed while others may succumb to the minor disruptions and conflicts. However, such complexity does not relieve either parents or social workers of the responsibility to ensure that children grow up in the kind of environment which is likely to provide opportunities for developing confidence, self-esteem, communication and inter-action skills, trust, the capacity for forming relationships, social controls and knowledge. In other words, the elements of affective and cognitive functioning which enable us to understand the world in which we live and to engage in appropriate social interaction with other people who share it ...

The book goes on to quote Kellmer-Pringle on basic emotional needs which 'must be met if children are to grow up into capable and confident adults'.*

It is, then, both professional principle and common sense that child care does include emotional and mental health care. If anything, indeed, in the social work literature, these elements are the core of child care.

However, it is not quite so simple!

* KELLMER-PRINGLE, M.L. (1975) *The Needs of Children*, Hutchinson.

Professional and Institutional Responses

It is one thing to say something applies at the level of professional and personal responsibility and in principle, and — unfortunately — quite something else to say it applies at the levels of institutionalized wisdom and practices. In other words, there is a world of difference between 'child care', as enunciated in professional literature, and 'residential child care' as a social service.

By 'institutionalized' I mean how practitioners (of any discipline or profession) behave when their holistic understanding of children's needs and their sense of personal responsibility towards meeting those needs, are compromised or circumscribed by professional and agency obligations, constraints or extraneous group loyalties (e.g. to trade unions or professional bodies), as well as by the practical difficulties of working with colleagues as a team.

Part of the institutionalizing process is inevitable once we recognize that child care comprises not only the adult-child (professional-client) relationship but also planned provision. Planned provision includes the setting in which personal care is provided — namely the planned environment or milieu which, if it is to be therapeutic, will become 'planned environmental therapy'. But planned provision also includes the managerial and administrative environment inside and beyond the specific service setting.

I think what I have just written is true even for fostering and adoption, which, in the earlier quotation, Carole Smith was writing about and — not surprisingly — preferring to residential establishments about which she concludes (on the basis of general research):

> Children may be handicapped in terms of learning social skills, developing an acceptable self-image and sense of self esteem, and attaining emotional maturity and stability.

All of this can happen in foster placements and with adoption, too, even where the relationships within the new family are understanding and caring. Foster parents and adoptors need support. Other services will need to be involved. In the case of emotionally damaged children, parents and children will need intensive support from outside in order to achieve the 'planned environmental therapy'. Such has been the intention, indeed, of professional foster schemes based on mutual and external support following the lead taken in Kent in the early 1970s. In such cases, and only on these conditions, fostering and adoption can be seen as therapeutic alternatives to the best that might be provided for some children (not all children) in a residential setting.

But Carole Smith was not talking about the best residential practice, but what, in general, actually tends to happen in a large number of residential settings. This takes us back to the question of what inhibits residential settings from achieving the professional ideals social workers espouse. How do we overcome our tendencies to behave 'institutionally' (e.g. bureaucratically) instead of in keeping with the best traditions of our social work or other professional background?

Some of the difficulties may typically come from restricted opportunities to train alongside other professionals working in the same field; from rules or set procedures; from fragmented systems of organizational accountability; from too many agencies tackling the same issues from isolated positions and from interdisciplinary and interagency rivalry.

Something we can do immediately, at a practical level, is to take time out from work to visit other establishments and to see how other people approach their tasks. This can help to free us from accustomed constraints. However, to apply what we gain from elsewhere to our own situation requires a right attitude to team-work, a willingness to allow us space to contribute to developing new practice as well as to have time to listen to our colleagues. This, in turn, requires there to be a congenial administrative framework — what Professor Chris Cullen, of St Andrew's University termed (in talking with me) 'a haven of administrative sanity' where team work will be effective.

When one thinks of the complex financial and organizational negotiations that have to take place to develop and run a residential school, it must sometimes be an uphill struggle. As

Chairman of Raddery's Council, I can recall moments of insanity. And Raddery, being an independent charitable company, is fortunately placed.

A Context for Inter-Professional Team-Work

How then, do we find this administrative haven of sanity where team work will be effective?

Broadly speaking there are two diametrically opposed ways of looking at staff interprofessional team work. The conventional way, in hospitals and in the community, is to think of specialists each with their own expertise which they apply separately to a group of people they are assessing, treating and caring for. In a classic form, this represents the traditional approach to medical and paramedical specialisms. Furthermore, there is a hierarchy of professional disciplines and a pecking order within each profession. This sometimes leads to unnecessary divisions within the medical fraternity. For example, epilepsy is a major concern of psychiatrists, neurologists and pharmacologists — each looking at the problem in an entirely different way. We can add to this the different training of clinical pyschologists, occupational therapists, nurses, social workers and others who would be concerned with epilepsy. The problem of developing an integrated approach becomes formidable. Furthermore, though it is less true perhaps now than, say, thirty years ago, each of the groups in their separate ways tend to be doing things TO patients and FOR patients instead of WITH patients.

The alternative approach is based on the philosophy of the therapeutic community. Let me illustrate this with a contrasting example from a hospital setting, namely, the therapeutic community setting of Dingleton.

The therapeutic community model of team work Maxwell Jones developed at Dingleton Hospital in Scotland (and earlier at the Henderson Hospital in London), recognized all professionals — and that included anyone with a contribution to make — as equals. There was no hierarchy or pecking order. This did not mean to say there was no leadership. Maxwell Jones himself was a charismatic leader and he encouraged leadership in others.

Professional team work was based on mutual support with each person contributing to a pool of knowledge and practice which their unique background, including training, experience and personality, offered. Finally, expertise took into account knowledge and participation of the patient himself or herself and their network of relatives and friends.

I visited Dingleton Hospital several times when Maxwell Jones was there, and since. Much of the day was spent in meetings when the various professionals, sometimes including the client and sometimes without the client, sat round in a circle. I remember a patient being asked why she thought she was in hospital. Her reply was 'to get better and to help other people to get better'.

The therapeutic community at a residential establishment for children includes the child as a contributor to the healing process of others. The evidence for this at Raddery comes from some of the entries in the children's diaries we considered in Chapter 4. Yet 'shared responsibility' in a therapeutic sense has limits where children are concerned, because, as David Dean pointed out (see page 44, Chapter 3) children also have a right to be cared for in a way which would not be applicable in a residential setting for adults.

Summary of Raddery's Contributions

The argument I have been putting forward in this chapter so far has been about applying the idea of the planned environment, humanized in terms of a therapeutic community, to residential child care settings including community homes and even supported fostering and adoption. There is much to learn from the Raddery experience in this respect. For example:

1   The integration of education and care within a holistic approach, for example at daily meetings.
2   The relatively non-hierarchical staffing structure (compared, for example, with most local authority structures) and the alternative functional roles of 'enveloper', 'focalizer', 'team leader' and so on.

3   The emphasis on communication and support amongst all of the staff and the avoidance of a junior staff 'sub-culture'.

4   The emphasis on 'connecting' with children and thus avoiding the negative effects of a children's sub-culture.

5   The richness and variety of activities to engage all aspects of children's potential and not simply dealing with problems.

6   At the same time not avoiding problems — dealing with issues as they arise, within an overall individualized programme and plan.

7   Attention to all aspects of a planned environment — from lighting to food, from 'venues' to animal-keeping, from art and music to counselling.

8   An emphasis on consensus and harmony wherever possible.

9   Recognition of the spiritual worth of each person and the practical expression of spiritual values underpinning other aspects of child care, for example, in morning meeting.

Crisis Intervention with Families at the Point of Referral

One principle of the therapeutic community, as practised at Dingleton Hospital, is not practised at Raddery. This is the application of a crisis intervention approach by the school at the time a child is referred.

To understand this in the Dingleton context, one should mention that the therapeutic community idea developed parallel with the discovery of modern drugs to control mental illness. The approach by the use of drugs, or at least a reliance on the use of drugs, was as far as possible rejected at Dingleton. The alternative approach was based on intensive group work stemming from the experience that mental health problems were derived partly from within the family and the community and not only within the patient. This meant in practice that when, for example, a doctor referred a patient to Dingleton there would be first of all at least one meeting to consider which group of staff should visit the family — perhaps a social worker and psychiatrist, or psychiatrist and nurse, or perhaps all three — and they would then visit the family, insist on seeing both partners (and perhaps the doctor as well) and start their therapy there and then. The result of such crisis intervention was that admissions dramatically decreased. The admissions ward was eventually closed and the superintendent's house became the new location for admissions.

I have described earlier (Chapter 2 and Chapter 4) some of the ways in which Raddery maintains contact with the parents and seeks their support. Some of the staff at Raddery would like to go a lot further in working intensively with families. The restraint is the limitation of resources. Some other member establishments in the Charterhouse Group possibly spend more time than Raddery in this field but none of them, so far as I know, has yet fully explored the potential of the therapeutic community approach in this direction.

Because of the 'who does what' traditions in child care (in its broadest true meaning), the referring agency is usually the education authority's child guidance service. Joint referrals with social work agencies may become more common. Often, much work has been done with the child and, sometimes, with the family before the referral is made. But this approach is still tending to see Raddery, or other residential placements, as the point of admitting past failures rather than as the starting point for intensive inter-agency work with the child and the family. In this case, the therapeutic community approach would extend beyond the residential establishment to the agencies working with the family. This notion would be in line with John Tollon's idea of what he calls an 'educative community' extending from Linnwood Hall to the community outside (see page 129, Chapter 5).

We know from the accounts of the Raddery children that this is needed. We know that the fortunes of the children while at Raddery depend — beyond anything the staff are doing — on what is going on at home. The progress of David (page 81), Warren (page 84) or John (page 94), for example, in Chapter 4 illustrated this. Agencies may be 'in touch', but this is not the same as getting a hold of the family situation and working with it within the concept of a therapeutic approach to the needs of the family as a whole — including the child who is absent much of the time at Raddery. The contribution from the therapeutic approach at Dingleton to this process is in seeing the referral point as one for crisis intervention, mobilizing all the resources the family and the professionals can offer. The result, granted enough input at this point, might be that some children, once referred, would never reach the stage of admission. And for the others, who do start, it would provide the shared framework for future child and family therapy.

Chapter 7

Special Education

Integration

Discussion in many countries about special education is currently dominated by the issue of integration. The debate is becoming polarized. The Centre for Studies in Integration (in London) argues that there are no children with special needs who could not be integrated into ordinary schools. In a recent BBC interview, Seamus Hegarty was asked:

'Are you saying that there shouldn't be special schools?' He replied:

'We're saying that this should be a long-term goal'.

He went on to quote examples from Canada where 'local communities can do without separate special schools ... where any children with any disabilities you want to think of are included in the mainstream with appropriate support'. He then added: 'That makes ordinary schools really very different places'.

Two American writers, William Stainback and Susan Stainback, go further and talk about a stage 'beyond integration'. They write about 'inclusive schooling':*

An inclusive school and the process of inclusive schooling
is the ultimate goal of the integration and mainstreaming
process. Once inclusive schools and inclusive schooling

---

* STAINBACK, W. and STAINBACK, S. (1990) *Support Networks for Inclusive Schools*, Brookes.

are achieved, integration and mainstreaming will no longer be necessary since there will no longer be anyone left to be integrated or mainstreamed.

Many of the proponents of integration put their arguments forward as part of a social movement, a campaign. Its target is what are seen as bureaucratic authorities who insist perversely in blocking parents' attempts to get their disabled children into ordinary schools and who, instead, insist on sending them to 'segregated' special schools. In this country, the local authorities and the government are accused of not putting sufficient resources to back the legislation of the early 1980s which, they claim, promised integration.

The problem with a social movement of this kind is that everything and everybody get blanketed together in sets of slogans, demands and obstacles about a single-question issue — 'segregation' or 'integration'. We certainly need movements and we need campaigns, but, in this case, we need to understand the complexity of what we are talking about.

I wonder if it is more likely that communities which are said to have achieved 'inclusive schooling' are those where some children are already excluded through channels other than educational channels? I am sure Dockar-Drysdale's 'unintegrated' children are to be found not only in the beautiful surroundings of the 300-acre estate at Cotswold, but on city streets, and in psychiatric wards of hospitals, prisons (yes, there are children in prison, even in Britain!), or in other 'special establishments' outside the ordinary education system.

Most of the research which has attempted to evaluate integrated versus separate schooling, or mid-points between the two, has focused on children with physical or mental disabilities (or both). Much of the evidence points towards the social benefits of integrated settings, though there are complications — at least so far as parents are concerned — for children with severe and profound learning difficulties (mental handicaps). A question I put to myself when I began to study Raddery was how far the evidence would support the same arguments for emotionally damaged children?

The answer I have found, as a result of looking at Raddery

and other residential schools for emotionally damaged children, is that the question needs re-phrasing. A question about 'What sort of school setting?' begs the more fundamental question 'What sort of residential environment?' In the case of Raddery, the holistic approach to education derives from the child's need for holistic care.

So the first question to be asked about Raddery children is not 'Which sort of school should they attend?' but 'What residential care setting do they need?'. The answer is that it is a therapeutic community setting which incorporates a very special approach to education.

As one of the Raddery staff members put it:

> Classroom teaching is a form of therapy ... At Raddery emotional and social difficulties lead to learning difficulties, not the other way round.

Our starting point, then is not 'separation' or 'integration' in relation to 'ordinary school'. This is an important 'second' question, certainly — as we saw for children like Zoe (see page 58 Chapter 3) — but the first question is about a residential therapeutic community setting. The question is whether the child who has suffered emotional damage needs to be cared for and educated — in the widest senses of these terms — in a single environment.

Let us apply this to the needs of some of the children we have discussed in earlier chapters. Could Zoe, for example, have attended mainstream classes without having to go to Raddery in the first place? What about Jamie, now at Strathallan? Could his needs have been met at an 'ordinary' school? It is too easy an answer to say that they were, in fact, NOT met in 'ordinary schools' — and even with extra support in those schools. Let us look carefully at what would happen.

The question for the teacher of an integrated class is whether individual discrimination can be sufficiently exercised to meet such diverse social needs as, for example, Jamie would present alongside all the others. This is not as simple as giving extra attention to a child with a more conventional 'learning difficulty' in an integrated class (either through a support teacher or by a class teacher). The main social task of such a teacher is to help the individual child to behave more appropriately, while helping others in the class to continue to be tolerant. But for Jamie and the others, the social learning required in the class-room (and out of it) was much more sophisticated and, even assuming the problems of disruption to others could be coped with, it is not clear what the effects would be of drawing in normal children to say Jamie's world of daily experiences. (I hope Jamie and his parents will forgive me for using him as an example. Jamie has made such progress at Raddery that we are talking in his case about the past, not the present.)

A friend of mine, Fiona Harkes, who is a teacher and who has worked with me on many research projects, suggested I should acknowledge at this point some of the problems the teacher faces. She listed:

Class size (vital!)

Pressure to prepare children for the next class (where another teacher may not be so interested in an individual approach)

Lack of home-school contact (a not insurmountable prob-lem given headteachers with vision)

Tradition

Insufficient time available in basic teacher training to pre-pare teachers for meeting special needs of children

Fiona continued: 'To overcome these problems would require a revolution in our education system, but you are talking about revolutions!' Then she added: 'The result of such a revolution would be to improve the education system for all our children not just for Raddery children and children in other specialist groups'.

A general paradox about residential special schools is relevant here. On the one hand, their future is called into ques-tion by bodies like the Centre of Studies in Integration. On the other hand, historically, they have been the source of inspiration and pioneering not just for children with special needs but for education in general. Special methods have been developed which have had much wider application. This is especially true in the case of schools for children with emotional difficulties.

People with special needs (adults as well as children) make us all think more deeply about the services we provide. For example, the simple cassette we use in our tape recorders was first invented for use with blind people who could not handle the more difficult reel-to-reel mechanism. Many features of education at Raddery are potentially transferable to the ordinary school and are likely to enhance educational opportunity for many other children at ordinary schools.

Raddery's Transferable Assets

Let us look at some of the transferable assets of Raddery.

The spiritual dimension to Raddery might be considered transferable. If the kind of Morning Meeting that David Dean has developed with his staff suits Raddery, why should it not suit an 'ordinary school'?

Morning meeting at Raddery is the foundation of the human bonding that characterizes staff support, staff commitment to children and perhaps (though this is difficult to know) the capacity of children to help one another at the deepest levels. This is not necessarily to argue for the precise form of Meeting, nor is the spiritual dimension to education solely expressed in such Meetings, whatever their form. What one can say, is that if the ordinary school is to become 'special' in the kinds of ways which would address the children's total needs, they could look to the Raddery experience for a lead. The details about 'how' must depend on the tradition of the particular school.

The concept of holistic education at Raddery springs from this commitment. In other words, education which does not recognize the spiritual dimension is not whole. It has a cornerstone missing.

I stated in Chapter 3 that holistic education at Raddery had length, breadth and depth. The 'length' means twenty-four-hour availability for educational input. The 'breadth' means responding to each and every aspect of a child's potential. The 'depth' means the involvement of the whole person, beyond the conventions of normal professional teaching, with another person who is seen as potentially a whole person. Such would be Raddery's definition of the teacher-child relationship, which could be an inspiration to any school.

Some aspects of the philosophy of the therapeutic community are transferable. This does not necessarily mean that the ordinary school needs such a complex set of meetings. The transferable elements might include the approach to teamwork and staff support, the involvement of children in the some of the management, relationships with parents and other professionals, and so on. It is really about the sharing of human resources and leadership.

These seem to me to be the main general assets which Raddery has which are, in principle at least, transferrable to an ordinary school dealing with children presenting, as Seamus Heggarty put it 'any disability you want to think of' alongside any other child.

The next question is whether and, if so, how the specialist components of Raddery (and other schools described in Chapter 5) could be transferred, along with these general assets, to the 'ordinary school'. Let me take the Foundation Unit as an example.

In its educational provision, Raddery adopts what is very much a child needs-led approach. The establishment of the Foundation Unit is a good example (see page 54 Chapter 3). It was conceived and developed for the specific educational needs of a known group of children. When these particular children grow up and leave Raddery for all one can tell it could be disbanded — though this seems unlikely because others with similar needs can be expected to follow.

The underlying question such a specialist provision raises is how effectively an 'ordinary school' could respond to such identified needs. There are, perhaps, two quite separate issues here. The first is about numbers. The second is about flexible planning.

Raddery takes forty children from all over the north of

Scotland and some from further afield. A proportion only of these have been identified as the children requiring the highly unusual facilities and resources of the Foundation Unit. The facilities include easy chairs, sofas, provision for messy activities and toys — such as sets of lego — as well as carefully planned lighting. Not all children even at Raddery need the kind of therapeutic educational approach to be found here. The chances of more than one or two such children in any 'ordinary' school class needing these things at any one time would therefore seem to be remote. Perhaps what would tend to happen in practice in an 'ordinary school' is that the emotionally damaged child would find himself in a special unit alongside the child with the 'nearest to similar need' to be eligible for an approach at this level. This might, for example, be an older child with profound learning difficulties or, perhaps, a very much younger child with mild difficulties. Whoever it was, it would not be a case of 'integration' unless — at a school that had already gone much further down the road to 'inclusive education' — there was no special unit of any kind. Here an emotionally 'unintegrated child' (to use Docker-Drysdale's terminology) would be sitting in a class of 'integrated' children. The management problems might well be insuperable and the interaction with other children would be possibly without benefit.

This is not to say that an individual teacher with vision and commitment in a congenial setting could not go a long way. To quote Fiona Harkes again:

A child who is emotionally upset due to major upheaval at home may be unable temporarily to cope with formal schoolwork. A 'Foundation' type provision could be more appropriate for a short time. Ideally, this should be provided without necessitating her withdrawal from the class and classmates. The teacher's ability to manage this is likely to be hampered by the number of children in the class. But in a small class, where the teacher is already using individualized programmes, it may be possible. Experienced teachers intuitively adapt their curricula content to cope with the temporary needs of children under emotional stress. Perhaps greater guidance in teacher training would help them to do this in a more structured way.

She pointed out it might be easier in a primary than in a secondary school setting.

The second question is whether the planning procedures of local authorities could match Raddery's capacity to respond to children's needs quickly enough to provide the necessary facilities, like a Foundation Unit, for which there had been a newly-identified requirement? In the case of Raddery, the requirement was recognized in July and — over a holiday period — it was ready for use in September. Furthermore, since the technical expertise came from within Raddery to plan, choose, purchase, modify and furnish the new premises, its tailor-made match to needs was assured. Are our 'ordinary schools' going to be able to do this?

An underlying theme here is that where we are dealing with children with 'very special needs' (and I am not now only thinking of emotionally damaged children) a 'second best' in educational terms is not good enough. This is a theme which runs through not just Raddery but New Barns, Cotswold, Linnwood Hall and the other schools compared with Raddery in Chapter 5. This is also a theme which gets beyond and behind the debates about the integration of children with special needs into mainstream schools. There is no disagreement about the argument for adequate staffing and other resources — neither 'inclusive' nor 'special' provision for children with very special needs should be provided 'on the cheap'.

Working with Parents

I want now to return to the integration issue from a different perspective, namely working with parents. In spite of its large catchment area, most parents or other carers travel to Raddery several times a year (for reviews, for the annual gathering, or sometimes just to pay a visit). The school staff also visit the families. Again, as with the arguments about integration in class, it is not the fact of contact with parents that counts but the professional purpose and depth of understanding that go with it. A school aiming to integrate emotionally damaged children would surely need trained social workers (or staff with dual teacher/social work qualifications as suggested by Warnock) within the school in addition to the senior school staff taking a personal interest in the children's home circumstances?

Another point to note is the flexibility of arrangements for individual children at Raddery to enable them to spend more, or less, time at home according to their needs and wishes at any given moment. In other words, the amount of home contact the child can either tolerate or gain from, is strictly controlled within an overall ongoing assessment and plan. How is this control effected from within the setting of an 'ordinary school'? Nothing less than the wider integration of education and social work services would be required (as Lord Kilbrandon in Scotland and others in England and Wales have, in the past, actually proposed). That, at the moment, seems a remote possibility!

In short, ideas like integration or 'inclusive schooling' cannot simply be introduced at the fall of a barricade (real or imagined!) at the doors of an ordinary school or education authority. The ideas have to take root in fertile soil and then begin to grow.

I would not like to pronounce absolutely in the meantime that the minimum educational needs of at least some of the Raddery children would not be catered for in some very exceptional 'ordinary schools'. I am saying even this would be incredibly difficult. It would not necessarily be the best way of providing the social education that is needed and, furthermore, even social education within a holistic framework is only half of what Raddery offers.

What about the residential setting? More importantly, what about the integration between the school and the residential setting? These questions must take us beyond the 'ordinary school' and what most people understand by 'education', so perhaps I should leave them for my final chapter.

There is another question, however, that does belong here in this chapter. Let us suppose you are an ordinary teacher in an ordinary school and you find a child like.... (I won't suggest who from Chapter 4, you can take your pick!) in your class.

What should you do? Some of the accounts in Chapter 4 suggest that teachers in some cases may even have tried to meet the child's needs from within the school for too long — and even that child guidance services may have struggled with the family problems for too long — before the child was referred to Raddery. I suspect other therapeutic communities would sometimes feel the same way.

There are two problems about a referral which is late. The first obvious one is that there is less time to work with the child and the family — and, indeed, probably less time for eventual integration into mainstream schooling from Raddery, where this is appropriate. The second reason is that the longer the referral is left, the greater will be the sense of starting from a situation of 'last resort' with its connotation of the 'disposal' of the child and of his problems.

I argued in Chapter 6 that a neglected facet of the therapeutic community approach to child care is the effort put into working with the child, the family and others involved at the time of the referral. This must include the 'ordinary' school, and the class teacher in that school. It would be nice to think that there could be a direct carry-through from the ordinary class-teacher to the Raddery teacher — and then back again to the ordinary teacher. This, if I understand it rightly, is part of the vision of John Tollan at Linnwood Hall in particular. Then, special and ordinary school together begin to constitute, along with others, the 'educative community'.

This is surely a more fertile field for discussion than a dogmatic argument about whether or not everything can be done for everyone within the 'ordinary' inclusive school?

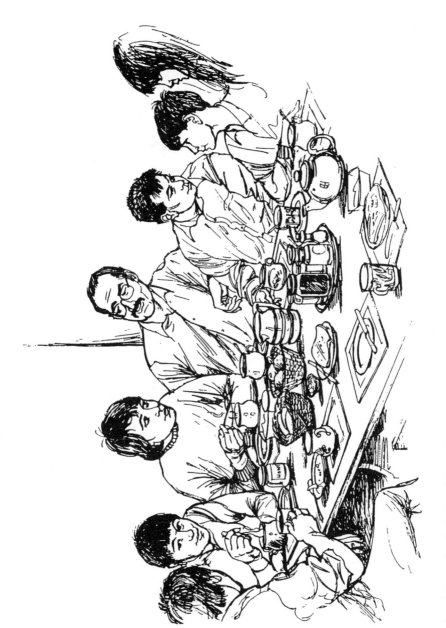

Lunchtime at Strathallan/weekly meeting.

Chapter 8

Preparation for Interdependent Living

By the time a Raddery child reaches Strathallan he or she is expected, firstly to have gained some useful insight into his or her past and present problems and, secondly, to be able to control his impulses sufficiently to relate to others on the basis of potential adult interdependence.

Assuming children who come to Strathallan meet these criteria, there are correspondingly higher expectations of them than at the main school. In particular:

1   More is expected of children at Strathallan in taking decisions for themselves.

2   There are higher expectations in terms of working together.

3   Children are expected to learn practical skills of management in daily living — cooking, tidying, shopping, and so on.

4   Children are expected to take some part in local community, activities.

At the same time, the setting still offers a large measure of protection and support and the expectations of the children are compatible with what they have been used to at Raddery. They are still part of the Raddery community. They attend community meetings at the main school (as Paul's and Jonathan's diaries showed). Some may be engaged on work experience at the main school site. Their attachment to Strathallan is something additional — but it is a continuing part of the care and education that Raddery seeks to provide.

Work at Strathallan is highly complex. There are, perhaps, three main groups of methods. The first is individual counselling. There appears to be more time for this at Strathallan than at the main school. The second is through role-modelling in a situation where there is close day-to-day contact in domestic situations as well as in wider social situations in the community. The third is through meal-time house meetings when domestic or social problems are discussed. In addition, as I said earlier, youngsters at Strathallan share the therapeutic community experiences of Raddery. There are also the same arrangements for reviews.

During the recent Raddery 'Community Week', when staff were gathering together and preparing for the coming year, one staff member remarked that Strathallan was a 'half-way' house, but that half way to 'what' was an open question.

For a few children, like Zoe (see page 58, Chapter 3) Strathallan provided support in returning successfully to normal schooling. For Paul (see page 71, Chapter 4) it provided an opportunity to gain in confidence — a path that was to lead to returning home and attending a Further Education Course. For John (see page 94, Chapter 4) it is helping him to face an uncertain future in the community, building on his creative potential. In talking about the aims of half-way houses, or similar ventures, emphasis is usually given to promoting 'independent living'. I have never liked this phrase, with its connotations of self-sufficiency, perhaps even self-seeking. It suggests learning to manage without depending on others. If followed too literally it puts an undue emphasis on the physical and technical aspects of coping. In a proper context, these are important. Learning how to open a can of beans without cutting your finger can be useful! But learning to get along with others in an adult world is more fundamentally important. (I accept that they are related — to develop practical skills may be a means to helping others as well as to helping oneself.)

The truth is that we all depend on others and others depend on us. Adulthood is about inter-dependence, not independence. A half-way house is about the specific stepping stones from a one-way dependence — where children are dependent on adults who are responsible for their care — to a new situation where they will grow into a state of adult interdependence with other adults. The same is true for half-way houses for adults leaving long-stay institutions. In this case, 'de-institutionalization' is part of a re-educative process to gain experience of adult-to-adult interdependence.*

In other words, the education provided at half-way houses, Strathallan included, is essentially social education. It offers experience of relationships in a new context — the context of adulthood and the interdependence this implies. Yet for Strathallan and Raddery children, the pathway to adulthood — even if everything has gone well for them — will not be straightforward.

This was illustrated for me when I showed Martin Macdonell, the Principal Assistant at Strathallan, what I had written about adult interdependence. He said, 'Yes ... I agree up to a point but ...' The 'but' consisted of the following:

> Interdependence is difficult for youngsters still at Raddery where they go home at weekends and where they have little to go back home to. In some respects they are still very dependent (loyal) to their families even when their chronological ages would imply that they should be able to move on.

He added:

> They may have effectively become alienated from family, school, friends and their communities by being at a residential school for most of the year.

The implications of these comments, if they are true, are serious. Granted that the children have to attend school in a

---

* See SEED, P. (1988) *Towards Independent Living*, Jessica Kingsley.

special residential setting in the first place (and this was the conclusion reached in Chapter 7), Martin is implying there is a social cost.

Adult 'interdependence' pre-supposes a stage of increasing 'independence' from home and parents as a part of growing up. Martin is saying that being at Raddery complicates this process, apart from the inherent difficulties the children will have anyway on account of their past experiences.

I would be inclined to think it is the emotional difficulties from the past which the children face which are the most important. If the first stages of being an adult — the processes of early adolescence — are delayed because of the problems the children have had to cope with, it can be argued they will be complicated because of the reality that the child (i) only goes home intermittently, and (ii) is likely to have mixed feelings about 'home' and parents anyway, which are established well before adolescence.

For a variety of reasons, Strathallan can only hope to go part-way with the youngster towards an adult 'interdependence'. Work must continue after the child has left Raddery and left Strathallan — and left home — even though he or she may be an adult in terms of chronological age only.

The social services often fail to provide for children leaving residential special schools or other residential establishments. There is a tendency to let the child flounder and then, when he is freshly labelled as offender, drug addict, homeless or whatever, new forms of 'adult services' or 'community care' come to the rescue. The continuity of care is often lacking.

An example in Scotland of a very positive approach to picking up past problems, once young people have been rendered homeless, is Glengowan House in Glasgow. This provides what its 1990 Annual Report calls 'a comprehensive and holistic service to the most vulnerable group among the growing number of young homeless people'. As a project of the St. Vincent de Paul Society, this venture tries to address the spiritual as well as the social and practical needs of the young people. The Report refers to 'the challenge ... to preserve the basic values of Christianity which are brought to life in the whole approach. These build up a sense of community while responding to the dignity and freedom of the person. They also accept the challenge to tackle issues of social injustice together with the young people who have suffered from them'. The Report analyzes the previous history of these people. Out of twenty-one, fourteen had suffered physical child abuse and eleven child sexual abuse. Sixteen had suffered family breakdown. Nine were described as having mental health problems. Sixteen had drugs or other solvent abuse problems. It is interesting that of the twenty-one, ten had previously been in children's homes, five in List D schools (equivalent to English community homes) and three in special schools.

The Report says 'During the past eighteen months there has been a steady demand for places at Glengowan.... With the present rate alone another centre could be opened tomorrow'.

Glengowan's experience confirms and illustrates the evidence I have gathered from Raddery and other special schools in two respects. Firstly it confirms what I said in Chapter 5 about the backgrounds of more severely emotionally damaged children finding their way into residential child care of one kind of another, and about the continued need for residential special schools which adopt a holistic approach. Secondly, it exposes the dichotomy and the gap between services for children and services for adults. In the Raddery context, it brings us back to the question, what lies beyond Strathallan?

There needs to be something after a 'half-way' house, and before young people experience homelessness and its associated difficulties. At the individual level this is part of the notion of 'outreach' which Strathallan is developing. It is interesting that in some areas it has been found that ex-Raddery pupils form their own local groups and networks. Outreach in this case means finding and facilitating local means to support such groupings rather than necessarily maintaining direct contacts.

We now can return again — and at a deeper level — to the question 'half-way to what?' The underlying question is whether the child has the potential during the time he is at Strathallan to develop into a 'good enough' adult to live interdependently in the community. If so, the fulfilment of the specific practical objectives which Strathallan sets for these youngsters will enable them to do so. Zoe, for example, will be reintegrated into normal schooling and everything else she has learnt at Strathallan should enable her to function well enough in later life. If, however, a child is still at an earlier stage of development during their time at Strathallan, on account of the extent of earlier emotional damage, they will not be able to develop sufficiently to survive when they leave without additional support and perhaps additional therapy. In this case, 'half-way' may mean 'half-way' to fresh opportunities for support and therapy as an adult.

A similar concern has led the Peper Harow Foundation and the National Children's Home to establish The Cumberlow Community in London. Melvyn Rose explained that this will be a new residential treatment centre for very disturbed young people (over the age of 16). After they finish a three to five years residential treatment programme they will move to a programme of continuing treatment in the community.

Not all Raddery children will be able even to reach the Strathallan stage. Some will still lack even the potential I have described. They may still be too self-centred, for example. They may be still be unable to sustain any relationship.

For these children, even a half-way stage to adult interdependence cannot be reached until they leave. For them to be able to make progress, everything I have said about treatment and support after leaving are all the more important. In such cases, continuing protection may also be needed — protection for themselves and sometimes for others. Ideally, within an environment offering a measure of protection — in other words this will often mean a residential setting such as Cumberlow Community in London and some existing provision from bodies like the Richmond Fellowship — therapeutic work will continue.

Of course the settings in which people live will determine what is demanded of them as adults. Certain kinds of settings will provide a 'let-out' from facing up to the full demands and implications of interdependent living. In military service settings, where orders are given and usually obeyed, where some forms of behaviour towards others are tolerated which might not be tolerated outside, where peer-group relationships are sustained on a limited basis while avoiding many issues that really matter, — in such a setting survival at an earlier level of

emotional maturity is possible and the demands of interdependent living in the community are postponed. They are
postponed until the time arrives for discharge.

Apart from this and similar escape routes, most Raddery
children are caught in the dilemma between various unresolved
needs from the past and realities of the present. On the one
hand, the realities of present family life are still a source of pain.
Yet because the child's emotional development has been interrupted he or she is not yet ready to think about moving away
from home. Their inclinations, on the contrary, are to gravitate
towards home, even if home is unsatisfactory.

Thus, at a time when children in more normal circumstances are thinking about distancing themselves from parental
influences, Strathallan youngsters are still searching for the
fantasy and warmth of an earlier home some never knew. It
is in this context that Martin's comments about the loss of
other friends in their local communities are pertinent. If youngsters do return home they may be doubly disadvantaged. They
have not an easy nor often even a feasible home situation to
return to. Sometimes they have not friends either in the home
communities.

When I shared these thoughts with Stuart Bates, another
member of the Strathallan staff, it prompted him to tell me the
story of a lad who had recently left Strathallan. His parents had
had psychiatric problems and at a fairly early age he had been
fostered. He had come to Raddery and progressed to Strathallan.
He had left as well prepared as could be expected. His foster-
parents offered a setting which was rich and compatible with
the richness of Raddery. From a superficial point of view, it
would have seemed everything was going for him in what his
foster-parents offered. Instead of being able to accept it, however, the first thing he did when he came of age was to leave
his foster-parents and return to his own parents. Here life would
be not only difficult but dull.

There is another factor here which some of the parents
pointed out to me. Many parents cannot be expected to compete
with Raddery in providing a comparable educational experience
and opportunity at home. In this context, Stuart suggested to
me, that some elements of Raddery were 'addictive'. Having

been at Raddery, children felt they needed to continue to have the amenities and opportunities that Raddery provided. By comparison, life at home was likely to be dull. If this is true while a child is at Raddery, it is also sometimes true for a child who has left Strathallan and returned home. Yet they are driven to return home.

There is a variation to this pattern in the case of some of the girls. Having a baby is not, in its early stages, dull nor, driven by instinctual behaviour, necessarily difficult. But as with joining the Services, this offers only a temporary — and much shorter — respite from the pains of growing up. As babies develop, they become demanding in more subtle ways and the involvement and responsibility on the part of mother is likely to require more thought-through responses. Angela was fortunate in this respect in so far as in the neighbourhood where she lived there was a close supportive network which she had not lost touch with (she came to Raddery relatively late). She was able to live a short distance away from her actual home and she received support from members of the extended family.

The importance of social networks in achieving the 'second half' of the process from 'half-way' cannot be over-estimated* Stuart drew my attention to a quotation from a textbook he was reading — 'Caring for Troubled Children' by J.K. Whittaker**:

> Residential and day provision for troubled children should function as a family support system rather than treat the child in isolation from family and home community.

Strathallan tries to hang on to that system where it can and when it can.

Half-way houses like Strathallan are not likely to have the resources to proceed far along the second half of the journey beyond what I have called the half-way stage to interdependent living. However, when children in Britain reach 18 they are

---

* For techniques for understanding and using social networks, see SEED, P. (1990) *Introducing Network Analysis in Social Work*, Jessica Kingsley.
** WHITTAKER, J.K. (1979) *Caring for Troubled Children*, Jose Bass.

eligible to benefit from the new provisions of the National Health and Community Care Act 1990. More specifically, some will benefit from the requirement to make plans embodied in the Chronically Sick and Disabled Persons Act — although all of the provisions of this legislation are not yet implemented.

But from April 1991, priority will be given to implementing part of the provisions of the 1990 Act so far as adults with mental health problems are concerned. As we argued in Chapter 6, mental health care is an integral part of good child care. Ex-Raddery youngsters should come within the provisions of the new Act in this respect, as adults in need of mental health care. The problem — as we said earlier — has been that society has waited for mental health problems to manifest themselves as gross social problems or difficulties before it reacts.

If the social services take to heart the intentions of the 1990 Act, this should no longer be the case. A needs-led pro-active approach is specifically advocated in the government's Notes of Guidance to the implementation of the Act.

It is true the legislators may have had in mind mainly older people leaving long-stay hospitals for whom care in the community may prevent the need for hospitalization. But Section 55 of the Act (for Scotland) states that 'for any person' for whom they are under a duty or have a power to provide, or secure the provision of, community care services, the authority:

(a) shall make an assessment of the needs of that person for those services; and

(b) having regard to the results of that assessment, shall then decide whether the needs of that person call for the provision of any such services.

This means in practice that, if local authorities will it, and are persuaded to give it a sufficient priority, they can provide, or secure other agencies to provide, community support — including, if necessary, residential and day services, for young adults along the second half of their journey to interdependent living.

Chapter 9

Return to Raddery and Summary of Conclusions

It is my final visit to Raddery to gather material. I am sitting in on one of the regular meetings of the 'envelopers' — the members of staff who have the specific responsibility to support others in the Raddery community. Spencer Houston — (Assistant Principal (Programme)) — is in the chair. It is late afternoon.

Time is very short. It has not been an easy day and much of it still lies ahead. Tomorrow the children go home for the mid-term break (Autumn 1990). Practical things like children's clothing have to be seen to. The agenda has not been completed and Spencer is trying to hurry the business to a conclusion. As often on such occasions, the meeting is in danger of wasting its last few minutes talking only about which items to discuss. Some people are visibly anxious to get away.

David Dean, sitting alongside the eight or so others, asks if he can have ten minutes of the meeting's time. The chairman replies 'No, not really'. Karen wonders if she and another member can leave and someone else will tell them what happened in their absence. David says he would rather everyone heard. Spencer says that David can have two minutes. David replies he will do his best.

David then reviews where the school is at, six weeks into the new arrangements involving different 'venues' and major new staffing arrangements. He likens it to a second adolescence for Raddery. It is easy for us to start fighting each other, at such a time he suggests — each one thinking about and wanting to promote their own particular interests. As envelopers, he said, our task is to hold the concept of the 'whole community together'. He mentioned that there were new members of the envelopment team and then he made a simple plea that envelopers make a point of being kind to one another, that they try to be nicer.

As usual, David holds the meeting by what he says and demonstrates the meaning of envelopment. A sense of confidence and attunement is restored.

To put this into context I should explain that, amongst other happenings, the previous evening all five boys from the cottage had absconded and spent the night rough in a village a few miles away. Strathallan staff and youngsters played a major part in rounding them up and bringing them back this morning. In the regular community meeting at two o'clock, David had spent about ten minutes saying what had happened and that he had decided that all five were being excluded. They had been sent home. They and their parents had been told they would have to re-apply in writing for a place, if they wanted to return. It cost a lot of money for a child to be at Raddery, he said, and if they did not want to be at Raddery, there were others waiting to fill their places. He said what had happened was nothing others should feel guilty about. The meeting then went on, with a quick change of mood, to all its other varied business — information and action points from the last meeting, problems, expectations and, finally, appreciations (of which there were many).

So it was 'business as usual' after the five most unintegrated boys in the school — for whom the cottage had been especially staffed and prepared — had absconded and been, temporarily at least, excluded. They included David and Warren, whose paths and progress we followed in Chapter 4.

Later, I clarified with David how the decision apparently to exclude the five children had been taken. Was it intended to be a bluff, I asked? David, pointed out that it had been meant seriously. But that it was the first time such a drastic decision had been taken. An exclusion was a very rare occurrence. One of the envelopers had sown the seed for the idea with reference to practice at another school. The idea then had been thoroughly discussed between David and Bill (Depute Principal), Mike

(Head of Care) and Eric (Assistant Principal, Family Work). David had also been concerned to gauge children's reactions — not by directly asking their opinions but by listening to their comments in discriminating betwen the children involved. They were perceptive in sorting out one child from another, he said. For example, they were supportive of Warren. They saw David (child) as a 'sheep'. We had to be involved, David Dean added, in what had been a sub-cultural trend which would repeat itself.

In this context, the main purpose of the exclusions was to demonstrate to the parents the statement that 'we work in a partnership of some depth'. In some cases, the parents had re-committed themselves and 'the experience was invaluable'.

I also learnt from one of the cottage staff that during the crisis, between the boys returning to school in the morning and their exclusion at lunch-time, some useful counselling had taken place. For example, one of the boys had been able to talk more openly about why he was at Raddery.

These events illustrate and perhaps express symbolically that there are neither simple conclusions nor easy answers in working with emotionally damaged children at Raddery. Nor can there be any easy simplication of the issues that the study of Raddery has raised. This would also hold true in other settings — in one of the other residential therapeutic communities, for example, or in the case of a social worker intensively working with a family, or a teacher, hopefully supported by others, in an ordinary school.

Be it the vision of a wider educative community, which is being developed from Linnwood Hall, or the intensive treatment approach at the Cotswold community, or the milieu of commitment to love and understand exemplified at New Barns, or the experiments in support schemes to ordinary schools — whatever the approach, there will be no record of smooth progress to the goals the staff, the children, the parents or the policy makers, have set.

But then, at the deepest spiritual level, the act of love is complete in itself. This does not abrogate the responsibility to examine methods and goals. But the testimony of effective understanding and care, as a method and as a goal — as the means and the end — rather than a search for what I have called 'smooth progress', is ultimately the yardstick of any 'success'. Those who work in this field are not in the business of doing things to inanimate or passive receptacles. Like parents, though not as parents, they are in the business of freely offering all the attributes of care and nurturing to those who find it hardest to understand what these gifts are or how to use them.

There is, then, in what I have seen and examined at Raddery (and more superficially elsewhere) a testimony to movement rather than evidence of 'smooth progress' towards desirable outcomes. We can apply this at several levels.

First, movement has taken place for each of the children we have considered. No-one has remained entirely 'emotionally stuck'. The children have moved on from where they were. They have not, in other words, remained untouched in the ways some of them appeared to be untouched in the schools they attended before they came to Raddery.

Secondly, movement has taken place in the development of Raddery during the time I have been writing this book. It has not, moreover, been the kind of typical institutional movement from an heroic start to a state of stable, routinized and dull respectability. Ten years after the start of Raddery, when I began writing this book, there was, perhaps, just a slight whiff of anxiety in something Alf said that this could happen. Instead, as David's phrase to the envelopers meeting suggested, I have witnessed a 'second adolescence', leading to a second coming of age.

Thirdly, there is movement in the way different schools and residential establishments which were hitherto often isolated are increasingly forging links. It is true there has always been some interflow of ideas, especially when staff have moved from one setting to another. But the pace has quickened and the dialogue has extended and become more disciplined and systematic. It is an international dialogue.

Fourthly, the context is now ready for a maturing to a deeper and wider understanding of community. We all need a sense of community. It expresses mutual support and commitment. The would-be closed community that draws its strength from hostility to other communities will give way to the more open community that grows as its vision broadens. For John

Tollan at Linnwood Hall, it is to an 'educative community' embracing local schools, clubs, parents, other agencies, and so on. Raddery, too, sees much of its future growth in terms of what it calls 'outreach'. This must be the way forward. The idea of envelopment must touch and ultimately include the community outside — including the 'ordinary schools' with 'ordinary teachers'.

I have suggested there are key points where this applies. The first is at the time of referral. The second is when the youngster, if accepted, arrives. The third is when they prepare to leave and after they leave.

I have further concluded that we should not think about referral, starting at Raddery or finishing at Raddery as fixed points in time. Obviously from an administrative and funding point of view, fixed points and periods of time are easier to cope with. But they are not the reality. Referral is a process which involves not only the current or previous school as an institution, but the class teachers and others in the school who are involved, as well as the child guidance service, the social workers and others.

This process should be recognized and used as an opportunity for preventative work. Perhaps one or two of the children might have remained in 'ordinary school' if enough community support could have been mustered. Perhaps one or two would have been better placed in other residential treatment settings if the referral had been seen more embracingly as a therapeutic opportunity for future work, rather than looking for a way out, for a 'disposal' of an immediate problem in a crisis. (I always think, what a give-away word 'disposal' is!). In this case, perhaps other children potentially more suited to what Raddery offers might have come. In any case, the children that did come would have come alongside on-going plans for working with other family members. This would probably have involved other agencies in the referral (recognizing that this introduces financial complexities, but also a more realistic commitment to care at home or at Raddery for all of the fifty-two weeks of the year). Such on-going plans have often been lacking.

The point that admission is a process is well taken at Raddery. We have seen that John's father was amazed not only to be shown round the school by another child but to discover the child actually liked the place! (see page 94, Chapter 4). I have been impressed by the care with which a new child is prepared for and received at Raddery. The idea of insisting on formally re-admitting children who have absconded re-inforces this point. Entry to the school is the process of developing a commitment to treatment and an undertaking to stick with it! It involves parents and children in a commitment to agreed goals.

The importance of the process of leaving Raddery is also recognized. It is also harder, not only because of lack of resources but because of its complexity. We discussed these in the last chapter in terms of preparation for 'interdependent living'. Again, John Tollan's ideas are very helpful. Indeed, when I showed him what I had written about Linnwood Hall for checking, he wondered whether I should place the piece in the chapter on interdependent living rather than in the chapter about 'other schools'. This, he indicated, was what Linnwood Hall was about. The important point is that the process involves an educative approach, or outreach, from a 'centre of excellence' to a whole range of resources in the community. This may, in some respects, represent an urban model rather than a model to suit the geography of the Scottish Highlands — but Raddery has a long way to go in developing, with other agencies, the full potential of an alternative or parallel development. In the meantime, the evidence suggests that some of the children return to a more socially and therapeutically impoverished environment, after the richness of Raddery, than could be attainable with more resources and vision. This might involve many other agencies working together on the basis that leaving Raddery or Strathallan is not so much an ending as a beginning (though it is rightly seen as an ending too). When all this is in place, in some cases, the leaving might take place a little sooner.

Finally, underlying all the movements I have described, I can discern a search for a deeper understanding of the needs of the children and of what the work is about. At one level, it is about more sophisticated theory linked to professional practice. At another level, it is about the words and the labels we use. I wonder whether society can wholly get away from euphemisms and ideologically loaded terminology?

Following the Warnock Committee report, 'special needs' became the terminology of schools and education authorities. The intention here was to individualize each child's needs, rather than to label children in terms of categories of disabilities. Meanwhile, until recently, social service authorities talked about 'handicaps' (most parents I meet still do!), but these have now become — in the case of mental handicaps — 'people with learning difficulties'. This terminology is supposed to signal a commitment to principles of 'normalization' or — even worse for the person who likes plain English — 'social role valorization'. In plain English, this means that a child's contribution to society should be valued.

The idea of a valued contribution to society, as a goal for children with special needs is an improvement on the goal of 'adjustment' which was implicit in the old label of 'maladjusted children'. Certainly, too, the Warnock insistence on individual needs is important and consistent with 'social role valorization'. Yet the problem with this approach to terminology is that it obscures the extent of the problems we are confronting when we come to consider the best education and care for the children we know about at schools like Raddery.

So a plethora of terms expressing degrees and kinds of special needs are coming back into fashion. 'Behavioural difficulties', 'severe emotional problems', 'profound learning difficulties', 'vulnerable', 'disruptive' and even 'unintegrated' convey all sorts of messages about the children they are intended to describe. 'Emotional damage' — the term I found at Raddery — has the advantage of distracting attention away from the children and onto the situations in which they have grown up and now find themselves.

There is, of course, an error in the opposite extreme of seeing children solely as victims. This is the starting point. They ARE victims — and society is the abuser, as well as often others closest to them. Many of them feel they have been abused in school and sometimes in a sequence of misplaced residential placements. But they, even as young children, are partners in movement in so far as there is that 'pocket of potential' as John Cross called it. The strength of the sophisticated theory I referred to — and I was thinking of Winnicott and Docker-

Drysdale in particular — is that, at its heart, is optimism. The 'unintegrated child' is differentiated from the 'psychopath' in that the latter term represents a psychiatric litter-bin, the former a dynamic offering of hope and worthwhileness. It was, incidentally, the psychopathic litter of a psychiatric hospital wing that Maxwell Jones picked up and began to work with in formulating the philosophy of the therapeutic community.

We discussed in Chapter 7 the extent to which aspects of the Raddery experience are transferable to the 'ordinary school' — to make 'the ordinary school special' as Tony Dessent terms it.* The question is whether the 'ordinary school' can ever be special enough for children who need an integrated residential and school placement on the therapeutic community model.

Perhaps it is the vision shared with the children, the commitment of staff to work together, and the shared community experience which are Raddery's most generally transferable assets to other places.

There are signs that the sense of community has reached its second adolescence and is coming of age in the wider world.

---

* DESSENT, T. (1987) *Making the Ordinary School Special*, Falmer Press.

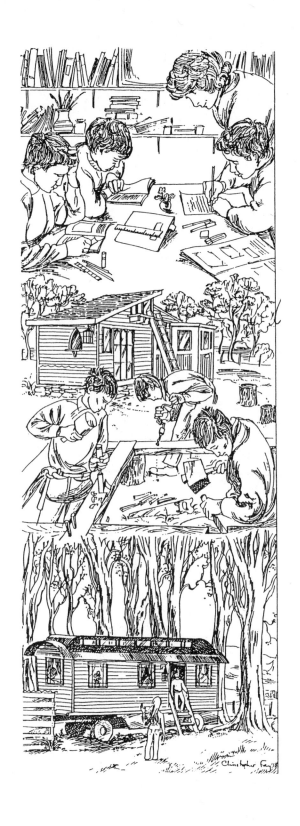

Index

Abbotsholme 16, 38
Absconding 14, 33, 176, 180
Adoption 2, 121, 145, 146, 147, 149
'Adrian' (staff) 72
Air Training Corps 77
'Angela' 78ff, 82, 102, 172
'Alison' 12
'Alleluyja' 67, 70
Amnesty International 67, 70
Animal-keeping 11, 36, 38, 55ff, 109, 150
Annual Conference 25
Annual Families Gathering 59, 70, 77, 83, 87, 160
Annual General Meeting 38
Art 52, 53, 66, 74, 84, 90, 109, 126, 150
Assessment 28, 31, 55, 63, 93, 124, 131, 148, 161, 173
Avoch 74

Badger, Bill (Depute Principal) 12, 14, 18–19, 36, 37, 48, 58, 82, 94, 176
Balbernie, Richard 111, 128, 136
Barnardos 137
Barns Experiment 4, 116
Bates, Stewart 23, 24, 172
Bedford Institute Association 116
'Betty' (Staff) 100

BBC Radio Scotland 60
Bicko, Steve 13
Birmingham University 19, 21
'Blowing in the Wind' 12, 13
Bodenham Manor 117
Borboro School, Uganda 17
Bridgeland, Maurice 107
British Association of Social Workers 145
Bruderhof 110
Bush, George 14

Camphill Movement 137
Carbarns, Eric 12, 19, 20, 23, 28, 106, 177
Careers Advisory Service 76
Cartref Melys 16
Centre for Studies in Integration, 153, 156
Charlotte Mason College 32
Charterhouse Group 108, 111, 123, 151
Child Guidance 4, 69, 76, 151, 162, 179
Children's centre 81, 86, 88
Children's Hearing 96, 97
Chronically Sick and Disabled Person's Act 173
Classes 1, 2, 13, 14, 18, 46ff, 63, 65, 66, 67, 68, 72, 73, 84, 85, 90, 91,

96, 97, 100, 101, 119, 120, 123, 124, 127, 155, 156, 159
Classes Meeting 38, 72
Clothing 52, 175
'Colin' 48
Colour 16, 34, 41, 50, 51, 52
Community care 2, 3, 168, 173
Community Meeting 14, 33, 34ff, 38, 39, 42, 59, 65, 66, 90, 165, 166, 176
Community Week 28, 166
Cooling, Maurice 128
COSLA 2
Cotswold Community 5, 25, 108ff, 121, 128, 136, 144, 154, 160, 177
Cottage, The (Venue) 35ff, 83, 87, 1099, 177
Council (See Raddery Council)
Counselling 18, 45, 46, 150, 166, 177
Craigerne School 137
Craft work 84, 115
Crisis intervention 150ff
Cromartie, Lady 40
Cross, John 117ff, 136, 181
Cullen, Chris 146
Cumberlow Community 170
Curriculum 51, 53, 55, 130, 134, 159

Daily Meeting 51
'Danny' 37
'David B' 36, 81ff, 89, 102, 151, 176
'David K' 49
Dean, David 5, 7, 14, 15, 16, 17, 19, 22, 23, 24, 29, 30, 38ff, 42, 43, 44, 51, 52, 55, 59, 60, 62, 63, 82, 87, 94, 120, 129, 134, 135, 157, 175, 176, 177
Dean, Valery 5, 7, 22, 23, 38ff, 57, Department of Education and Science 123, 127, 135, 144,
Dessent, T 182
Dick, Jim 25
Dingleton Hospital 148, 149, 150, 152
Disabilities 3, 181

Docker-Drysdale, Barbara 111, 115, 121, 154, 159, 181, 182
Drama 12, 49, 75, 77, 84, 85, 126
Duke of Edinburgh Award 132
Dundee University 142

East Quinton School 125
East Sussex CC 125
Elgin 14
Educational Priority Area 129
English 46, 49, 53, 62, 71, 75, 79
Epilepsy 148
Ethos 30ff, 53

Faith and Light 74
Families Gathering (See Annual Families Gathering)
Family Service Units 16
Findhorn Foundation Community 16
Focalizer 5, 38, 44ff
Fogell, Jon 125
Food (See also meal-times) 17, 17, 44ff, 68, 82, 101, 113, 150
Fortrose 6, 20
Fortrose Academy 58, 59
Fostering 2, 102, 121, 145ff, 171
Foundation Unit 1, 26, 54, 158, 159, 160
Fox, George 16
French 66
'Frozen' children 112, 115
Fry, Christopher 7, 78, 94, 99
Fund Day 37, 48

'George' 99ff
'Gerry' (Staff) 37, 74, 89, 99
Glasgow Remand Home 116
Glengowan House 168ff
God 14, 17
Gorbachov 14
Grace (after meals) 17
'Graham' 73
Grampian Region 2
Gray, Jenny 37, 50, 51, 52
'Greta' (Staff) 75
Gulf crisis 50

Harkes, Fiona 156, 159
Harris (venue) 26
Hegarty, Seamus 153, 158
Henderson Hospital, London 148
Highland Region 2, 6
HM Inspectors of Schools 18, 53, 54, 62, 125
Hodgkin, Robert 16
Holding (children) 113
Holly, Buddy 13
Homer Lane Trust 118
Hospital(s) 3, 92, 129, 148, 149, 150, 154, 173, 182
Houston, Spencer 55, 73, 75, 90, 175

Iceland 12
Inclusive Schools 153ff, 161
Integrated (children) 25, 54, 112, 115, 136, 176, 181, 182
Integration (with ordinary schools) 2, 3, 24, 58ff, 88, 136, 137, 141, 153ff
Inverness College of FE 99
'Isobel' (staff) 75

'Jamie' 66ff, 74, 76, 78, 102, 155, 156
'Jason' 72, 74
'Jonathan' 89ff, 102
'John' 89, 94ff, 102, 151, 166, 179
Jones, Howard 117
Jones, Maxwell 148, 182
Journal of Therapeutic Communities 113
Joyce, C.A. 110

Kanjuri School, Kenya 21
'Karen' (staff) 175
'Kate' (staff) 67, 73, 89
Kaye, Peter 132
Keenan, Colin 25
Kellmer-Pringle, M.L. 145
Kent (Fostering scheme) 147
Kilbrandon, Lord 161

'Lachlan' 67
Lancaster University 19
'Lee' 37, 42
Lenin 134
Leningrad School 12, 132
Lennon, John 14
Linnwood Hall School 129ff, 136, 151, 160, 162, 177, 179, 180
'Local Hero' 11, 12
Locheil Outward Bound School 32
Love 5, 13, 14, 15, 40, 59, 60, 117, 120, 144
Lubovski, Vladimir 133

McDonnell, Martin 23, 24, 167ff
MacGoveran, Pat 25, 50, 54
Main House (Venue) 26, 109
Makarenko, Anton 133
Manchester University 20
Mandela, Nelson 13
'Margaret' 46
Maths 53, 844, 85, 126
Maupassant, Guy de 49, 50
Meal-times (see also Food) 18, 26, 31, 41, 53, 85, 122, 166
'Michael' 46
'Mike' (staff) 176
Millar, Peter 111
Mochrie, Graham 83, 87
Moorclose School, Workington 19
'Morag' (staff) 91
Morning Meeting 2, 8, 11ff, 41, 63, 89, 111, 122, 150, 157
Mother Theresa 14
Mulberry Bush 111

National Children's Bureau 107
National Childrens Homes 170
National Curriculum 55, 126,
National Health and Community Care Act, 1990 173
Ncholenge School, Zambia 21
NE London Polytechnic 23
New Barns 115ff, 160, 177
Nepommashi, Yuri 134

North Wales 16
Nuffield Foundation 107
N.V.Q 55

Oak House, The 78, 84, 91, 94, 95
'Oliver' (musical) 77
Organisational analysis 28
Outdoor Education 16, 39, 54, 55

Parents 2, 3, 4, 6, 20, 53, 59ff, 66ff,
   103ff, 112, 118, 120, 121, 122, 125,
   126, 128, 131, 133, 141, 142, 145,
   151, 154, 156, 158, 160ff, 168, 171,
   176, 178, 179, 180, 181
'Paul' 66, 71ff, 102, 166
'Paul' (staff) 81
Peper Harow 25, 54, 144
Perth External Behavioural Support
   System 131ff
Planned environment 146, 149, 150
Playfield House 129
Poor, Dick 23, 24
Psychiatry 28, 86, 92, 128, 129, 130,
   135, 148, 151, 154, 171, 182
Public relations 60ff

Quaker (See also Society of Friends)
   111, 112, 116, 122

Raddery Council 4, 14, 22, 23, 25,
   38, 53, 62, 148
'Raddery Rag' 96
Radysh, Wolodymyr 137
Reid, David 52
Rainer Foundation 111
Referrals 2, 3, 21, 92, 119, 120,
   150ff, 162, 179
Robert Gordons Institute of
   technology 25
Research 4, 65, 194, 105, 107, 111,
   128, 146, 154, 156
Research Institute for Defectology
   133
Respite 24, 88, 122, 172
Reviews 20, 105, 106, 122, 128, 160,
   166

'Richard' 67
Richmond Fellowship 170
Rose, Melvyn 25, 144, 170
Rosemarkie 20
Rossie Farm School 116
Royal Air Force 86
Russia 12, 41, 71

St Andrews University 147
St Luke's College, Exeter 19
St Vincent de Paul Society 168
Satir, Virginia 34
Science 50, 53, 84, 96, 109
Scottish Office 18, 125
SCOTVEC 49, 52, 55, 63
Seed, Philip 167, 172
Selly Oak School 23
Sexual abuse 3, 136, 169
Sexual assault 33, 169
Shotton Hall School 32
Skye (Venue) 26
Smith, Alf 20, 21, 28, 30, 58, 67, 72,
   90, 178
Smith, Carole R 145ff
Smoking 41, 101, 102
Social Work 2, 3, 4, 20, 22, 23, 25, 28,
   53, 83, 85, 86, 117, 129, 142, 143,
   145, 146, 147, 151, 161, 177, 179
Society of Friends (See also Quakers)
   16
'Sofia' 100
Spence, Elizabeth 23, 28
Staff conference 31
Staff meeting 38, 58
Stainback, Susan 153
Stainback, William 153
Standard Grades 9, 55, 63, 96
Steiner Communities — See also
   Camphill 29
Stoddard, Ben 117
'Strangest Dream' 12
Strathallan 6, 22, 23, 24, 25, 34, 38,
   44, 45, 58, 59, 71, 72, 77, 89, 90,
   91, 92, 93, 97, 99, 102, 109, 145,
   163, 164ff, 176

Stratheden Hospital 129
Summer camps 105, 106
'Suzie' 58
Swalcliffe Park School 127ff

Teachers 4, 46, 52, 55, 62, 71, 83, 90,
  96, 104, 115, 117, 124, 126, 127,
  131, 132, 135, 142, 144, 156, 159,
  162, 179
Teacher's Meeting 38, 58
Team leader 29, 81, 87
Team-mate 14, 31, 81, 85, 99, 101
Teamwork 28ff, 104
Therapeutic community 1, 5, 15, 18,
  30, 32, 33, 38, 40, 41, 44, 108, 111,
  136, 137, 148ff, 155, 158, 162, 166,
  177, 182
Thomson, Margaret 6
Tidmarsh, David 29, 32, 33, 46, 49,
  50, 52, 58
Toddington 118
Tollan, John 129ff, 162, 178, 182
Toman, Mike 137
'Three-Way-Flyer' 12

Uniform (school) 62
Unintegrated (children) — See
  integrated.

Venues 1, 25, 26, 87, 127, 150
Volunteers 115
'Yvonne' 14
'Yvonne' (staff) 100

Warnock Committee Report 181
'Warren' 84ff, 102, 121, 151, 176,
  177
Western Isles 6
Whittaker, J.K. 172
Whitwell, John 111ff
'William' 37, 57, 100
Williams, Bryan 142
Wills, David 4, 111, 116, 117, 118,
  122,
Wiltshire CC Social Services
  Committee 110
Winnicott 111, 181
Winston House, Cambridge 116
Work experience 44, 45, 53, 71, 78,
  80, 97, 100, 126, 127, 128, 166
Wyndham School 19

Youth Hostels Association 128
Youth Training Centre 71
Youth Training Scheme (YTS) 93

'Zoe' 58, 59, 73, 155, 166, 169